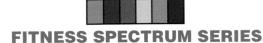

Fitness AQUATICS

FITNESS SPECTRUM SERIES

LeAnne Case
Aquatic Alliance International

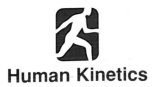

Human Kinetics

Library of Congress Cataloging-in-Publication Data

Case, LeAnne, 1958-
    Fitness aquatics / LeAnne Case.
        p.   cm. – (Fitness spectrum series)
    Includes index.
    ISBN: 0-87322-963-0
    1. Aquatic exercises. I. Title. II. Series.
    GV838.53.E94C36   1997
    613.7'16–dc20   96-369
                                                                                          CIP

ISBN: 0-87322-963-0

Developmental Editor: Nanette Smith; **Assistant Editor:** Henry Woolsey; **Editorial Assistant:** Coree Schutter; **Copyeditor:** Thomas J. Taylor; **Proofreader:** Erin Cler; **Indexer:** Joan Griffitts; **Text Designer:** Keith Blomberg; **Layout Artist**: Doug Burnett; **Photo Editor:** Boyd LaFoon; **Cover Designer:** Jack Davis; **Photographer (cover and interior):** John Guin—except where otherwise noted; **Illustrators:** Dianna Porter, line art; Studio 2-D, Mac art

Human Kinetics books are available at special discounts for bulk purchase. Special editions or book excerpts can also be created to specification. For details, contact the Special Sales Manager at Human Kinetics.

Printed in Hong Kong   10 9 8 7 6 5 4 3 2 1

Human Kinetics
Web site: http://www.humankinetics.com/

United States: Human Kinetics, P.O. Box 5076, Champaign, IL 61825-5076
1-800-747-4457 e-mail: humank@hkusa.com

Canada: Human Kinetics, Box 24040, Windsor, ON N8Y 4Y9
1-800-465-7301 (in Canada only) e-mail: humank@hkcanada.com

Europe: Human Kinetics, P.O. Box IW14, Leeds LS16 6TR, United Kingdom
(44) 1132 781708 e-mail: humank@hkeurope.com

Australia: Human Kinetics, 57A Price Avenue
Lower Mitcham, South Australia 5062
(08) 277 1555 e-mail: humank@hkaustralia.com

New Zealand: Human Kinetics, P.O. Box 105-231, Auckland 1
(09) 523 3462 e-mail: humank@hknewz.com

Contents

Acknowledgments

I would like to thank all those who have helped me in making this book a reality—My aquatic class participants, who let me practice all kinds of new and wild ideas on them, and who draw the best out of me with insightful questions and feedback. My children Chad, Kristin, Stephanie and Matthew who, at times, willingly cooked their own meals to give me a bit of uninterrupted time. My parents Gerald and Marilyn Sharp who raised me to believe I can do anything. My husband Jeff who is very supportive, and continues to park his car in the driveway, so I can store my water toys in the garage. Six great women, who also happen to be experts in various aspects of aquatics, who have taught me so much—June Andrus, Mary Essert, Pauline Foord, Lynda Huey, Jane Katz and Ruth Sova. My editors at Human Kinetics, Ted Miller and Nan Smith, who have shared their extensive writing abilities and been very patient, as I have completed this project during an intensely busy time. Most of all, my Father in Heaven to whom I am grateful daily for all things great and small.

PART I

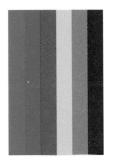

PREPARING FOR FITNESS AQUATICS

One of today's newest and most popular ways to exercise involves getting wet. More than six million Americans have chosen water fitness as their favorite form of exercise: People of all ages, sizes, and fitness levels have taken the plunge.

What is the all-around best form of exercise? Is it cross-country skiing, jogging, cycling, aerobic dance, or aquatic exercise? Whatever your answer, you are correct! Experts agree that the very best exercise is the one *you* can stick with and enjoy. With aquatic exercise you can pursue fitness in a backyard pool, lake, or public facility, and at a level that fits your personal needs.

Water fitness offers not only efficiency, comfort, safety, and fun, but also training at any level of intensity. Couples or friends at different fitness levels can work side by side, proceeding at their own pace. Athletes who are injured can maintain fitness while they wait to regain use of an injured body part. Water pushes back only as hard as it is pushed, magically offering gentle or intense workouts.

More than a set of exercises for jogging, jumping, or dancing around in the water, aquatic fitness is a specific science of movement with its own set of rules and a long list of advantages. If you are familiar with swimming, you know swimmers design every motion to streamline the body, helping it cut and slice through the water. Vertical water exercise has the opposite objective. Each motion aims to *maximize* resistance, creating turbulence, opposition, and drag to strengthen the body. The water can be a medium for aerobic conditioning or relaxation, low impact or no impact, fat burning or strength training. Any health benefit derived through exercise will happen faster and safer in the water.

In this book part I explains how you can use aquatic fitness to improve your health and increase your independence, having fun now and throughout your lifetime. You will discover much more:

- How water assists all areas of physical fitness
- How the properties of water can change the way you exercise
- What equipment and apparel choices will benefit you
- How to make use of your available water site
- How to evaluate your current level of fitness
- How to determine your *water-adjusted* target heart rate
- What body mechanics and techniques will best fit your workout needs
- How to warm up, stretch, and cool down

You can make enormous improvements in your physical and mental well-being with fitness aquatics. The biggest hurdle for most of us is simply making the commitment to do it. Part I lays the groundwork for your upcoming motivation and success. Read on!

1

Aquatics for Fitness

Do you remember the ancient legend of the fountain of youth and its miraculous waters? According to legend, one drink of the extraordinary liquid would renew vigor, remedy disease, ease pain, and even reverse the effects of old age. The story is true—with one exception: Youth and good health can be found not by drinking from the fountain, but by climbing right into it.

As you read this book, there are people in the water experiencing relief from pain, being energized, and receiving renewed vigor through their aquatic workouts. Nearly all their muscles are involved while working out in the water, yet any chance of soreness or pain is washed away. Like them, through fitness aquatics you can feel in control of your well-being as you set goals and achieve them.

Who Gets Wet?

Vertical water exercise requires no swimming skills, although it incorporates some of the same body movements. Nonswimmers may initially be a little afraid of the water, but their success and enjoyment of water exercise soon overcome the fear, and many of them add swimming lessons to their exercise regime.

If your lifestyle is busy, then you'll be pleased to learn how efficient water exercise can be. One gallon of water weighs 8.33 pounds, a respectable amount for just one hand to push. Consider that an average 37 pounds of resistance meets you as you swing one leg through water. Water's resistance varies according to depth and speed, which you can always control. You achieve fitness without soreness or injury that might slow you down or cause you to regress. Men and women, old and young, feeble and athletic, all are discovering fitness in the water.

Water-exercise success stories come from an array of organizations:

- Dallas Cowboys (NFL)
- Los Angeles Dodgers (MLB)
- Denver Nuggets (NBA)
- U.S. Olympic Track & Field Team
- U.S. Marine Corps
- Notre Dame University
- YMCA and YWCA
- Duke University Medical Center
- Canadian Armed Forces
- Cooper Aerobic Institute

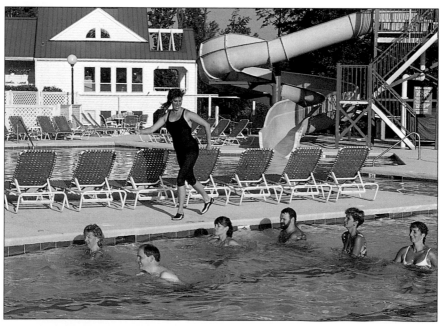

Vertical water exercise can bring success and pleasure even to the nonswimmer.

Why a Water Workout?

The physical laws of motion specific to movement in water state that eddy resistance occurs right behind the direction of movement as the water swirls and rushes to fill the space just vacated. Tail suction is another type of resistance: Water flowing past a moving part creates a current that slows movement down. Add a few waves and some frontal resistance from a flat nonstreamlined surface being pushed through the water, and you find yourself surrounded by a maximum workload.

In a recent study comparing the muscle mass of the heart among various collegiate athletes, water polo players and oarsmen were found to have the largest mass. Both activities involve working against the resistance of water. Many similar studies have brought to light the advantages of water fitness.

What to Expect From Water Exercise

Your body is a fine-tuned machine. With proper maintenance it keeps going and going. Regular workouts allow your body to perform the rest of the day's activities better. You can expect to reach farther, sleep more soundly, and move with more power and strength. Regular exercise improves your reaction time and alertness; balance and coordination improve as your brain, ears, eyes, skin, and muscle work in harmony. Let's look at other physical changes that occur during exercise.

Cardiovascular Benefits

Your cardiovascular endurance level indicates how well your heart, lungs, and circulatory system can deliver oxygen to the working muscles for a *sustained* period of time. Your muscles need oxygen to release stored energy. To increase the capacity of your heart and lungs, you must use large muscle groups in rhythmic, continuous motions—walking, jogging, swimming, clogging, bicycling, dancing, and water fitness workouts of all kinds—commonly referred to as **aerobic activities.**

All exercise programs are composed of three distinct components: *frequency*, *intensity*, and *time*. Each component is variable and allows you, a personal trainer, or a doctor to set obtainable goals:

Frequency refers to *how often* you exercise. Experts tell you to perform aerobic activities three to five times per week to maintain and improve your cardiovascular condition.

Intensity refers to *how vigorously* your body is exercising. Heart rate and exertion, two common ways to measure intensity, increase in direct proportion to how much muscle mass you are using.

Table 1.1
Benefits of Cardiovascular Exercise in Water

Muscle soreness virtually eliminated	LDL cholesterol and triglycerides lowered
Less stress on joints, muscles, tendons	Mind relaxed and rejuvenated
	Stress relieved
Stronger heart and lungs for increased energy	Self-esteem improved
Increased lean tissue and reduced body fat	Decreased risk of heart disease
	Increased alertness and positive attitude
Enjoyment	Everyone can participate
Nearly every muscle used in one workout	Work at your own pace

Time, of course, refers to *how long* you perform the activity. Big-time savings come in strength training and toning activities performed in the water, because they give the same results as land exercise in one-fourth the time.

Time and intensity work together when we talk about cardiovascular fitness. There are no shortcuts. You must work at your chosen heart rate for a minimum of 15 minutes. Water workouts described in this book keep you within your training zone for 20 to 45 minutes. It's a good idea to measure your intensity at each workout, to make sure you don't run out of steam before the end of your desired workout time, and to be certain you are getting adequate cardiovascular training. The heart muscle needs to be taxed enough to be challenged but not so much that it is overwhelmed. If you become overtired, you're more likely to perform the exercises poorly and waste time.

Muscular Strength

Current research suggests we are each born with a set number of muscle cells, which increase in size and strength when subjected to a *gradual* increase in workloads. To increase muscle strength, work the muscle at a level above what it usually experiences: the *overload principle.* Muscular strength is improved with a few repetitions at a heavy load of resistance. While under water, a muscle is surrounded by constant, multidimensional resistance—the deeper the muscle, the more resistance. After your workout, the muscle should feel fatigued, or gently tired. The *weight* of the water increases your strength. In time, if the weight of the water is no longer providing overload to your muscles, you can add equipment that increases the surface area of your arms, legs, or body, thus increasing drag and making you work harder as you move more water. Over time, your muscle will "rise" to the occasion and adapt to the new load it is working against.

The best news of all is that muscular strength is achieved 4 to 12 times faster in the water than in any land-based program. Sound too good to be true? Just try any of your favorite land exercises in the water. The sheer weight of the water will surprise you (and slow you down). Depending upon the depth of water and your speed, you will be moving 1 to 60 pounds of water!

Muscles work in pairs, referred to as antagonistic "muscle pairs." Successful weight lifters are careful to work a muscle on the back side just as much as its partner on the front side (i.e., the biceps and triceps, the quadriceps and hamstrings). In a weight room or exercise class, your muscle has resistance only as it pulls up against gravity. When under water, a muscle has multidimensional resistance; strength is increased in all parts of the muscle and all different joint angles, due to the constant resistance of the water as you progress a body part through its full range of motion. Ignoring muscle balance can increase the potential for injury, compromise posture, and create pain. Fortunately for aquatic enthusiasts, the water naturally balances the workload in any antagonistic muscle set (as long as equal force, speed, and resistance are given in both directions).

Muscular Endurance

Muscular endurance is the ability of the muscle to make repeated contractions with a less-than-maximum load. The muscle size will not increase noticeably, but the tone and energy level of the body will improve. Endurance exercises actually increase the number of capillaries that bring oxygen to that muscle. Endurance is improved by progressively increasing the number of repetitions required of the muscle group (i.e., swimming 10 laps this week, increasing gradually to 30 laps in four weeks, or three leg lifts today, progressing by one each day until you reach 20 lifts).

Body Composition

The human body is basically composed of two components: lean body mass and body fat. *Body composition*, the percentage of lean body mass compared to body fat, is more important than a person's actual weight.

Just what is a reasonable amount of fat? Today's society tends to judge fat harshly. Too much fat is unhealthy, but keep in mind that without

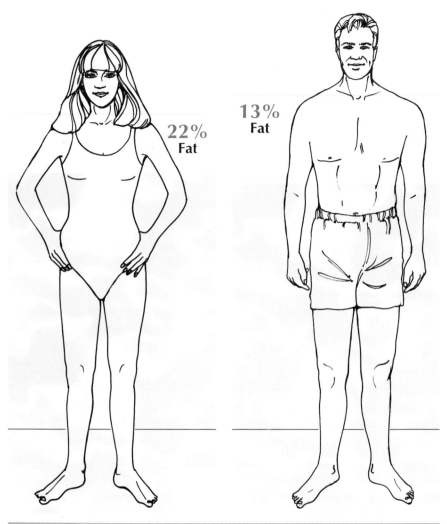

Figure 1.1   Your body by weight

some fat, we cannot survive. Fat stores nutrients and hormones, insulates our body, provides cushioning, and protects our vital organs. Body fat, for most people, fluctuates during the year according to seasons, holidays, and activity levels. Without an active fitness plan, body fat can increase as much as 5 percent per year.

When a person's weight is more than 20 percent above average for his or her body type, the benefits of fat become overshadowed by medical concerns. At this point a person becomes predisposed to conditions like diabetes, hardening of the arteries, bone and cartilage degeneration, and stress to the weight-bearing joints. Water is the safest place to exercise for people with any of these medical concerns.

Fitness aquatics is an excellent way to change your body composition. From any chapter, choose a workout that keeps you in your target heart rate zone (THRZ) for 30 to 60 minutes. Included in each workout will be an estimate of calories burned per hour. In the water, there is little trauma to the joints, less chance of overheating, and therefore less fatigue, injury, or discomfort, so you can work out even longer!

Fitness and Flexibility

Flexibility is the ability to move a joint comfortably through its full range of motion. Flexibility, which prevents injury and contributes to daily comfort through ease of movement, is influenced by age, activity level, health of the joint, and genetics. You can improve your flexibility, especially in the water, where flexibility often improves with little or no effort! The deeper you are in the water, the less you weigh. Water's buoyant effects reduce the pull of gravity, so every joint is less compressed, and every part of your body weighs less, yet you are supported and cushioned from every direction, freer to move in the water than anywhere else on the earth's surface.

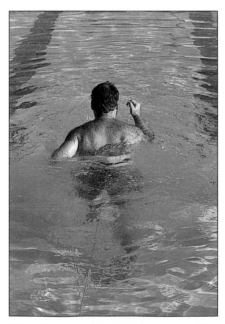

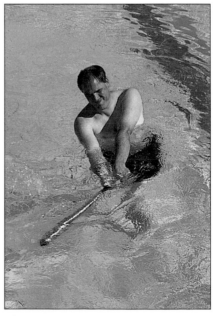

Six million people enjoy the safety, efficiency, and accessibility of water exercise.

Almost any activity can be enhanced with aquatics.

Balance and Coordination

Balance and coordination, which occur subconsciously for most of us, help you function more efficiently in daily activities and greatly affect your athletic performance. It takes your brain, eyes, inner ears, and muscles all working together to shift weight and evaluate spatial changes to keep you upright. The waves and weightlessness of the water stimulate the entire balance and coordination system. Aquatic exercise heightens and fine-tunes our movement sense with repetition and feedback in a very safe environment.

By now, you have at least an inkling of the fantastic impact fitness aquatics can have on your life. Water exercise is accessible to all, year-round, whether in a pool, lake, or ocean. Injury-free and highly powerful, water workouts are the most efficient use of your allotted fitness time. And if none of that impresses you, more than six million people agree: Aqua exercise is fun, pleasant, and invigorating! Let's get you equipped for some fun.

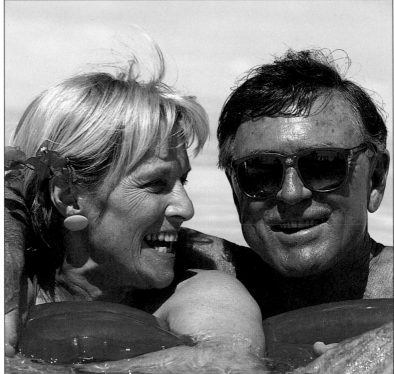

© F-Stock/ David Stocklein

Aquatic exercise is great for all ages and body types.

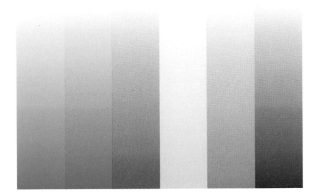

2

Getting
Equipped

The benefits of fitness in the water are no longer a secret. We are witnessing an incredible boom in the invention and marketing of aquatic fitness clothing, shoes, flotation devices, power-building products, pools, and private tanks. I've compiled a current and comprehensive list of water-specific equipment as well as tried-and-true tips, expenses, and information on shoes, swimwear, and some of the extra "fun stuff."

Where's the Water?

Anyone with the desire can find access to a suitable body of water. There are a few things to consider as you prepare to exercise in the water: What will ensure a safe environment? Which workouts are best in which pools? What's the best temperature? Let's find the answers.

Choosing Pool Depth

Mid-chest water is ideal for shallow-water exercising. Subtract 12 to 18 inches from your height to determine your ideal water depth for a shallow-water workout. At this depth, your body is protected from impact but still has enough weight and leverage to control your movement. If you have shallower water, you can make adjustments, like bending your knees or taking a wider stance to keep more of your body underwater, where it can reap the benefits. You may opt to do more work horizontally, holding the pool edge or using flotation in each hand, if the water is very shallow. The more your arms are in the water, the faster the upper body will respond to conditioning. Shallow-water workouts result in improved aerobic capacity, muscle tone, energy, and strength. Use your arms in the water at least 85 percent of the time.

Deep-water workouts usually require a minimum of six feet of water but, depending on your height and the amount of flotation you use, you could possibly get by with less. Just don't scrape your toes! Deep-water exercise generally implies that your feet will not touch bottom. Your head will be just above the surface, supported by your choice of flotation device. Deep water gives added resistance and protection to everything under the water. Many of the same exercises can be done in deep or shallow water. Deep water gives you more room to move your arms and legs in a full range of motion, allowing you to engage more muscle mass. Flexibility, strength, and endurance can all be increased very comfortably. If you are confident in deep water, imagine the ecstasy of a deep-water workout in the ocean, your legs whipping firmly against the weight of the water and the gentle motion of the sea. Give it a try on your next vacation at a lake or ocean.

SAFETY CHECKLIST:

- Never swim alone.
- Know the depth and temperature before jumping in.
- Water should be clean and free of obstacles.

Down Under

Pool bottoms are notorious for their slippery painted or tiled lane lines. Textured pool bottoms, on the other hand, can scrape the bottom of your feet. *Footwear* is the answer to these problems, as well as to slimy stuff often found on the bottoms of ponds and lakes.

You should be wary of sloped pool bottoms, because repeated exercise on the slope can cause posture problems and muscle imbalances. If there are no other places to exercise, be sure to change direction often so that each foot and leg share the slope time equally. Your other choice when faced with a slope is to use flotation and make it a deep-water workout instead.

Water Temperature

Shivering is an efficient way to burn fat, but it certainly is not pleasant. The average desired water temperature for fitness aquatics is 83 degrees F. One degree either way makes a noticeable difference. Those with a lower body fat or those focusing on flexibility and relaxation moves will prefer temperatures near 85 degrees. Those with their own insulation, or with plans for a high-intensity workout, usually prefer water around 82 degrees. Cool water requires a longer warm-up time because the muscles and blood vessels automatically contract to conserve body heat. Cooler water can be very invigorating. You are likely to move a little faster and give yourself a better workout if you also are trying to stay warm. Many swim teams keep their pool thermostat set at 78 degrees F. Anything much lower than that requires extra precautions.

You can lose body heat up to 20 times faster in cold water than in the air. If you always work out in cold water, invest in thin thermal swimwear specially designed to keep you warm. If the water is only occasionally too cold for your comfort, add a thin layer of insulation like a short-sleeved T-shirt, bike shorts, or leggings, to help hold in body heat. (Even socks and shoes can be worn if your toes bother you.) Layers should consist of fabric that will not weigh you down and that can dry quickly. Water will feel cool when you first enter because of the difference in body temperature and water temperature. Dress for how you will feel after the warm-up.

Burning calories means dissipating heat, and water over 88 degrees F interferes with the whole process. Exercising in warm water brings on greater fatigue, increases swelling, and accelerates blood flow. The heart beats faster (to cool the deep tissues) but not in a way that improves fitness. High humidity also interferes with the cooling process because it slows the evaporation of sweat, our number one cooling defense. Exercising in the heat can create medical emergencies. Don't risk it! Change your plan to a total-relaxation or deep-stretching session. Drink plenty of clear liquids before, during, and after you exercise. Try to find a shaded part of the water. Start early in the morning or late at night. If possible, end a warm water class with a three- to five-minute cool shower, constricting the blood vessels and returning the exaggerated blood flow from the surface to the core of the body.

At the Top

The higher the altitude, the less oxygen there is in your blood; your heart has to beat more times to provide the same amount of oxygen to the working muscles. If you find yourself traveling in higher elevation than you are accustomed to, work at a slower pace in order to train at the same target heart rate (THR).

Well Suited

You may have all that's needed for aquatic fitness already in your closet, or you may soon be doing some shopping. Here are a few things to look for as you decide what to wear in the water.

Swimwear

Did you know that 81 percent of all swimwear sold never hits the water? Much of the swimwear available is designed for sun bathing, and is made of less expensive fabrics. Reputable manufacturers who supply swim team or fitness suits use the better fabrics that last longer and save you money. Whatever kind of suit you choose, look for chlorine-resistant Lycra fabric. In some instances, what you decide to wear might not be a traditional swimsuit. Bike clothes, dance wear, or shorts and a t-shirt can be used. Most anything goes, as long as you're free to move. Some, but not many, pools today with antiquated filtration systems prohibit street clothes; just to be sure, call before you get wet for the first time. If you attend an established class, cultural norms may decide what you wear. The latest trend is bright-colored clothes that are psychologically stimulating and easier to see in the water. Professional instructors are usually clothed from head to toe expressly to contrast with the water, so their clients can better see what they are doing. When you add bright-colored shoes, bike shorts, and so on, a coach or instructor can see your motion more clearly and better help you with proper form and technique.

Swimwear should allow freedom of movement and yet offer support. Try the suit on and move in every direction you expect to move in the water. You should be comfortable moving in all directions. Females need enough fabric to support the bust: double layers of fabric, smaller armholes, or high backstraps. Males seem to prefer suits that are less restrictive yet not so bulky that they fill with water and swish around. Many swim trunks have built-in athletic support.

Sole Support

Designed to be worn in the water, aqua shoes provide traction which gives you stability and (if you desire) the chance to be aggressive. Shoes give your feet support, and protection from small abrasions. With the extra measure of protection from shoes you can concentrate more on intensity and form. Look for a shoe that fits very snugly around the ankle or that can be tightened while still dry. Once wet, all shoes tend to loosen up. Any shoe you choose should be worn only in the pool and surrounding areas; shoes worn on asphalt, dirty cement, and so on, bring foreign materials and chemicals to the water that counteract with the pool environment. If you are in the pool every day, consider two or more pairs of shoes. Wet shoes tend to develop mildew and bacteria. All shoes last longer if rinsed with fresh water before and after entering the pool. Shoes range in price from $6 to $60.

Eye Protection

You will need goggles for workouts that include swimming laps. They make the view clearer and give some protection from chemicals and bacteria. Always try before you buy! One eyepiece pushed against your eye socket should create enough suction to stay there a few seconds. All goggles should be made of soft, flexible materials. Silicone seals and gaskets are best. Goggles range in price from $2 to $10.

Wearing glasses for a workout is fine. Wear contact lenses *only* if you have no plans to go under the water. Contacts often get lost, and all lenses are affected by chemicals and bacteria in the water. Most doctors suggest even waiting 15 to 30 minutes after a swim to put contacts in, to allow your eyes time to cleanse themselves completely of pool water. Prescription goggles range from $10 to $150; unless scratched, they will last indefinitely. Rinse goggles before and after a swim to protect the elastic and the factory-applied anti-fog applications.

Heads Up

Some people wear swim caps to keep hair out of their face, give team association, or make a fashion statement. Lycra caps are water-permeable, inexpensive, and useful for holding earplugs in place. Caps of rubber or silicone, when fitted properly, can actually keep your ears and hair dry. You can expect to pay $3 to $5 for a basic cap, or in the $15 range for custom logo or fit.

Skin Deep

Any time your aquatic fitness routine is outdoors your skin is at high risk for skin cancers from direct sunlight and ultraviolet reflections off the water surface. Avoid any trouble by using these simple precautions:

- Use water-resistant sunscreen, SPF 15 or higher.
- Wear sunglasses with 100 percent UV protection to shield your eyes and reduce tension from squinting.
- Wear a thick shirt to cover any skin not well under the water.
- Wear a wide-brimmed hat or visor; a scarf can protect your neck.

Equipment

Try some new equipment in the water—for fun, variety, safety, intensity, or just for adapting to unique situations. You can use equipment for aerobic training, for strength and toning, for increased flexibility, or just for relaxation. Your equipment choices fall into three categories: buoyancy, resistance, or weight. Products that give you buoyancy or increase your resistance in the water are effective and efficient, but I suggest staying away from weighted products unless you have a specific fitness project in mind that requires them. Some products—Gyrojoggers, barbells, and kickboards, for example—can be both resistive and buoyant. A word of caution: Water is a safe place to exercise—until you introduce something that alters the governing principles of the water. Be sure you use the equipment correctly and safely.

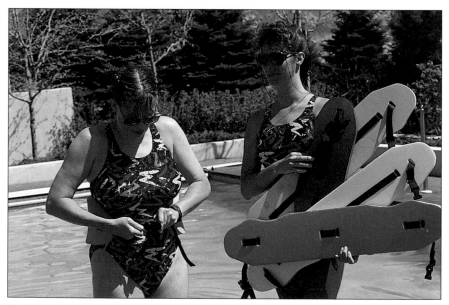

Used carefully and correctly, a buoyant belt frees your lower body for uninterrupted motion in deep water.

In deep water, a buoyant belt frees your lower body for uninterrupted motion, allowing you to increase your range of motion and work a greater muscle mass. Since you don't have to worry about keeping your head above water you can really focus on posture and technique. Buoyant hand or ankle equipment also gives you a lift, by increasing overload to that extremity. Because the force of buoyancy always pushes up, the workload is unequal; you will work hard pulling the arm or leg down, and have lots of help letting it move up. To maintain a balance between muscle pairs, return slowly and in a controlled fashion. Don't let equipment "pop" up to the surface.

Resistant equipment will increase the amount of water you displace. The greater the surface area, the more resistance. Fins, hand paddles, Hydro-Tone boots and bells, webbed gloves, and kickboards all increase the surface area as you push and pull them through the water. Some of the most popular aquatic products used for resistance include Aqua blocks and bars, Gyrojoggers, kickboards, hand webs, and Hydro-Tone accessories. The following list describes each product in more detail.

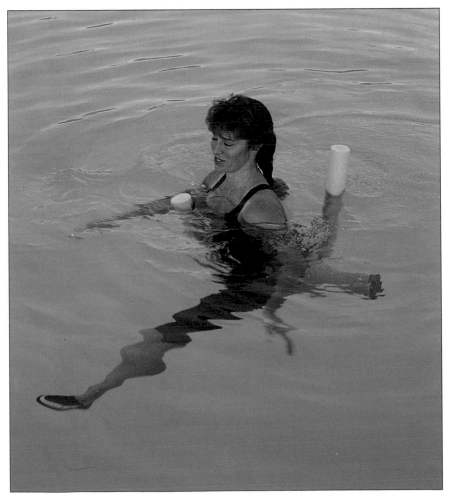

Water Woggles increase resistance and buoyancy.

Aqua Blocks

Aqua blocks, small barbells made for the water, increase the resistance as you press your arms through the water. They also can be used for flotation as you work the lower body or just relax. It is best to start small and work your way up to the larger sizes as needed. Aquatic Foam Accessories makes two sizes with add-on buoyant foam pieces, allowing you to work at just the right intensity and progress toward more resistance in increments; they are available at $25 per pair.

Flotation Belts

Flotation belts have become highly engineered, due to advances in aquatic science. Ask these questions when purchasing a belt: Is it thin enough on the sides that your arms move freely in a natural position? Are the abdominals exposed or unrestricted enough to contract effectively? Is it comfortable? Does it hold you high enough and in a balanced vertical position? Your choices among flotation belts include A.F.A. Waterap ($30–$45), J&B Foam's Water Walker ($7) or Aqua Deep Wrap ($12–$13). Bioenergetic's Wet Vest I and II are available for $60 and up. The Aqua Jogger, by Aqua Jogger Water Workout Gear, costs about $50.

Gloves

Hand webs are gloves webbed between the fingers to increase resistance and drag in the water, used by both swimmers and vertical exercisers to amplify the power of each stroke. Some manufacturers have webbed gloves that inflate! Hand gloves are not suggested for people with severe arthritis in the hand; the hand benefits more from the increased blood flow caused by water circulating between each finger. The neoprene glove from D.K. Douglas is $20 per pair, and comes in your choice of six bright colors. Hydro-Tone's workout glove is silicone ($20 per pair).

Gyrojoggers

Gyrojoggers, the most versatile aquatic product available, consist of two circles of foam, one inside the other. Used in deep water and shallow, they are designed to fit around the feet or the hands. Soft cell foam makes these so comfortable that you hardly know they're there. They can be used with no grip or a loose grip. Add, subtract, or adjust the foam pieces to vary the resistance. They really save you money because you can do so many things with them. Gyrojoggers are about $35 per pair.

Hydro-Tone Aquatic Exercise Equipment

Foot-worn Hydro-Boots and hand-held Hydro-Bells amplify the resistance of the water while promoting muscle balance, endurance, and equal-strength ratios. Hydro-Tone aquatic systems are lightweight, nonbuoyant, and easy to use.

Kickboards

Kickboards are found in almost every aquatic environment and can be used in many ways. All boards are not the same, however. Look for very rigid boards to give the drag and resistance needed for water workouts. You will need two, one under each arm, if you participate in deep-water exercises. A favorite, made by J&B Foam, is thicker than most boards, easier to grip, and healthier for the joints. This board gives great resistance and is buoyant enough to support most people for upper body work or races! Prices range from $6 to $15 each.

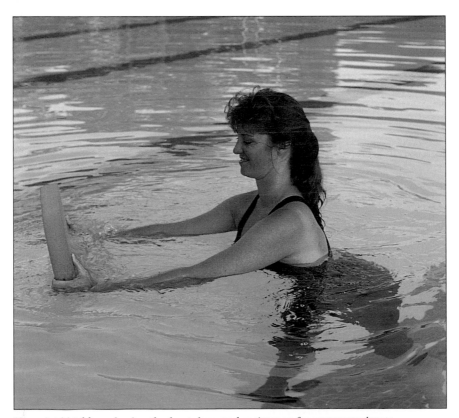

Very rigid kickboards give the best drag and resistance for water workouts.

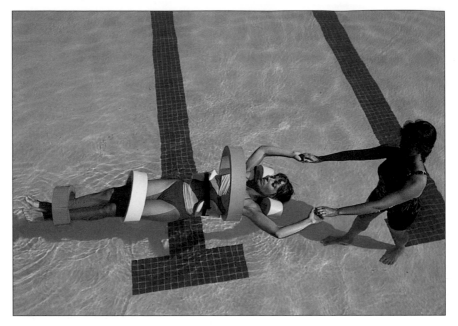

Body hoops are loved by all for relaxation, therapy, or swimming lessons and they rest inside each other for easy storage.

Aqua Step

Yes, step aerobics has been taken to the water! Water reduces the impact to the joints, heightens the resistance for multidirectional moves, and keeps you much cooler. Your beats per minute will be slower in the water and the moves are altered slightly to maximize buoyancy and drag. Make sure the step will not move around under water. Prices range from $60 to $90.

Water Woggles

Water Woggles are the hottest foam product currently on the market. Sit on them, lie on them, hang on them, push and pull them, straddle them, or tie them in a knot. Woggles are a 4-inch cylinder of foam, great for resistance, flotation, or stability, that support the weight of children and adults in deep water or shallow. Water Woggles are used as bicycle substitutes in water-only triathlons around the world. Available in four bright colors at $7 each. Quantity discounts are available in boxes of 20.

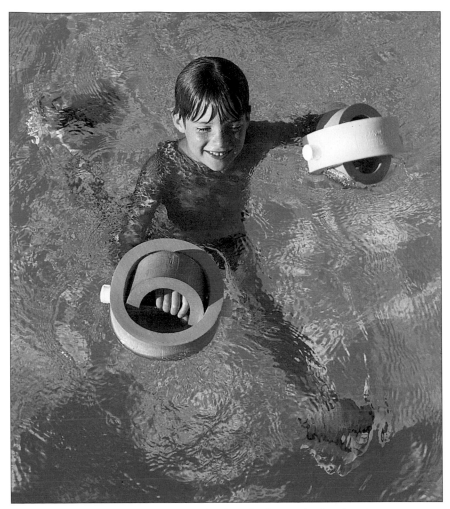

Gyrojoggers are designed to fit around either the feet or the hands.

Wet Wrap and Wet Pants

The neoprene wet suit vest designed by D.K. Douglas Company, with overlapping design that is easy to put on, gives you a custom fit. Indoors or out, the wet wrap, wet pants, and mock turtleneck provide warmth and sun protection without interfering with your full range of movement. The wet wrap can actually extend the length of your workout time in cool water, or extend the season in outdoor pools; it's available in six wild and wonderful colors for children and adults. Prices, based on size, range from $26 to $70.

ADDING UP THE COSTS

How much you spend will depend on what you already have, and whether you prefer only essentials or like some extras.

```
LOW-BUDGET COSTS
SWIMWEAR                          $    15-30
WATER SHOES                            10-15
SUNSCREEN                                  5
AVERAGE COST                      $    30-50
```

You can spend more for high-quality swimwear and equipment.

```
HIGH-BUDGET COSTS
SWIMWEAR                          $    30-75
WATER SHOES                            25-85
SUNSCREEN                              10-15
FLOTATION BELT                         25-60
UPPER-BODY EQUIPMENT                   20-60
LOWER-BODY EQUIPMENT                   30-100
AVERAGE COST                      $  140-395
```

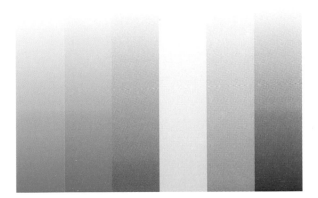

3

Checking Your Aquatic Fitness Level

You can't get where you're going if you don't know where you are. Evaluating and charting your changing fitness level will help keep you healthier and motivated by giving you a way to measure your progress. Self-tests (included here) help you determine strengths and weaknesses, thereby enabling you to devise the best plan of action.

First, complete the participation checklist to determine if you may proceed without a physician's approval. Next, choose one or all of the self-tests; the results will let you know where to begin. You will accomplish more in the long run with an honest fitness appraisal at the start.

Participation Checklist

Water is the safest place to work out. Before beginning any new physical activity, it is best to consult with your doctor. If you answer "yes" to any of the following questions, consult your physician before proceeding with any water exercises.

1. Do you smoke more than 10 cigarettes a day?

2. Do you suffer from chest pains or pressure, fainting, or severe dizziness?

3. Have you recently recovered from surgery?

4. Are you taking any prescription medication?

5. Will this be your first exercise in many years?

6. Do you have any chronic pain, bone, or joint problems that may be aggravated by exercise?

7. Has a doctor ever diagnosed you with heart problems, diabetes, or high blood sugar?

8. Are you pregnant?

9. Are you 30-40 pounds overweight?

10. Are you over 45?

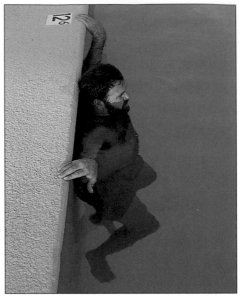

Stretching on edge of pool

Testing Your Limits

The following self-tests will help you decide where to begin your workouts. Test yourself again in six to eight weeks to see how you have improved. You will notice that these fitness tests measure the basic fitness principles discussed in chapter 1. You also may notice that these self-tests are all performed in the water! This idea is new territory because, traditionally, most athletes or patients are tested and assessed on land and then given a water workout prescription. Many health experts around the country, questioning why the water could not be the testing medium, have established alternative water tests and standards.

Testing is influenced by a variety of factors—water depth, medications, concentration, amount of sleep, types and time of food, temperature of the water and air, and humidity. To be accurate, take care to equalize as many factors as possible from test to test. Testing will be easier and more accurate if you have a partner who can count or time your movements.

Cardiovascular Test

Every time you test you will get a better feel for how it should be done. As you re-test you will see a pattern of improvement over the months. One recent study at the University of Texas, Dallas, found that inactive adults measurably improved their heart function after just 12 weeks of aquatic aerobic training. Here are two ways to test your cardiovascular strength, one of many factors that contribute to a healthy fitness level.

THE 500-YARD RUN

This cardiovascular test has been developed at Ball State University, Indiana, to measure aerobic conditioning.

1. Determine the length of the shallow water you will test in, and calculate the number of lengths required to cover 500 yards (20 lengths in a 25-yard pool).

2. Measure the depth of the water on your body so you can create identical circumstances next time you test.

3. After a basic warm-up, run 500 yards in the water as quickly as possible.

4. Record your finish time to the nearest second, and your heart rate.

5. Cool down in the pool and stretch.

6. Compare your numbers with the table below.

If this test leaves you extremely breathless, unable to talk, faint, or dizzy, please seek medical advice before proceeding. Common sense should tell you if you have overexerted yourself.

Table 3.1 500-Yard Water Walk/Run Norms		
	Males	**Females**
Excellent	<6:47	<7:58
Good	6:48-7:30	7:59-8:38
Average	7:31-8:14	8:39-9:19
Poor	8:15-8:57	9:20-10:00
Very poor	>8:58	>10:01

Notes: The symbol < means "less than" and the symbol > means "more than."

Norms are for people under 30 years of age.

Muscular Endurance Test

This test was developed by Juliana Larson, a personal trainer and therapist, in Eugene, Oregon. Her husband, as well as all foresters, must have an annual physical fitness assessment to maintain their position on the force. To keep things as accurate as possible, note water depth and any other details so you can reliably reproduce the same test later.

In deep water with a flotation belt, or in shallow water standing in place, jog as fast as you can. Have a partner count how many times your right knee raises up in 30 seconds. Standing in shallow water, perform a double biceps curl as many times as possible in 30 seconds, again counting one side only. Record your results for comparison in six weeks.

Body Composition Test

You might record your body weight before you embark on your fitness aquatics program, but because muscle weighs more than fat you will notice changes in musculature before weight goes down. Someone trained in the use of calipers, electrical impedance equipment, or hydrostatic weighing can measure body composition in a number of different ways. In his book *Fit or Fat*, Covert Baily mentions a quick way to "guesstimate" your lean vs. fat. Try to float in the water. If you sink slowly even with your lungs filled with air, you are most likely less than 20 percent body fat, a ratio expected for a fit male and for an athletic female. If you float with ease you are probably higher than 20 percent body fat, which describes most adults.

Flexibility Test

The support and density of the water makes flexibility testing in water much safer than on land. As always, use proper form, and if there is any discomfort, stop.

- **Finger touch:** (Shoulder) Try to touch your fingers behind your back with one hand going over the shoulder and one hand under the shoulder. Measure the distance or overlap between the middle-finger tip of each hand. Switch arms and record both numbers.
- **Straight leg raise:** (Hamstring) With your back and hips against the wall, raise one leg straight in front of you. Hold this position while a partner measures with a yard stick how far off the bottom you have raised your leg. Change legs. Record your results.

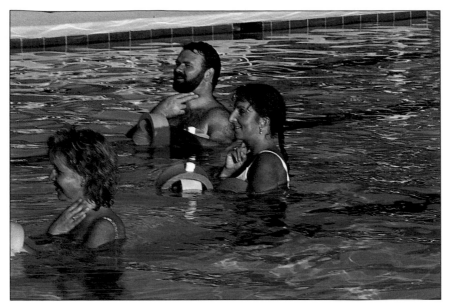

Monitoring heart rate

Monitoring Heart Rate

One way to measure the intensity of your workout is by heartbeats per minute. Within the range that your heart is capable of beating, there is an optimal window of opportunity. Much like the miles per gallon of a car, your heart receives maximum cardiovascular benefits within your target heart rate zone, or THRZ. This zone is different for each person, depending on age, fitness level, general health, and fitness goals. It is worth the effort to compute these figures. Your heart muscle needs to be exercised, just like the other muscles in your body. As your heart becomes stronger and more efficient, it can actually pump a greater volume of blood with each beat. It becomes better at delivering oxygen to the muscles, so you soon notice (among other things) that your working and resting heart rate will go down! Resting heart rates are very accurate in suggesting your current level of fitness. A strong heart beats fewer times to pump the same volume of blood—a sure sign that your aquatics fitness program is working well!

Completing step #5 on the following page gives you your personal suggested water-adjusted THR range. During actual exercise, it's best not to stop cold! While still in motion you can take a representative sample of what the heart is doing. Hydrostatic pressure of the water slows your heart rate before you can finish counting a 60-second heart rate check. You will get a more accurate reading of your HR intensity by counting

Step 1: You need to first know your heart rate at rest. The best time to check your resting heart rate (RHR) is in the morning before you move out of bed and before the alarm goes off. If that is unrealistic for you, try counting your pulse when you have been sitting very quietly at rest for 20 to 30 minutes. Simply find your pulse and count the number of beats for 60 seconds. If you find your RHR is greater than 100 beats per minute, please consult a physician before exercising. Record your number in a safe place for future comparison (e.g., RHR = 60).

Step 2: Predict your maximum heart rate (MHR).

MHR = 220 - your age (e.g., 220 - 30 = 190).

Step 3: Determine your heart rate reserve (HRR) by subtracting resting heart rate from maximum heart rate.

HRR = MHR - RHR (e.g., 190 - 60 = 130).

Step 4: Determine your target heart rate (THR).

Multiply HRR by the desired intensity. This is usually between 55% to 85% of MHR. If you feel that you have a very low fitness level or you have a limiting health condition, you may start your workouts as low as 40% intensity.

(HRR x 55%) + RHR = Lower range of target

(130 x .55) + 60 = 72 + 60 = 132

(HRR x 85%) + RHR = Higher range of target

(130 x .85) + 60 = 111 + 60 = 171

Between these two numbers is your target heart rate zone for land-based exercise. Remember these two numbers for cross-training on land.

Step 5: Subtract 17 from both the lower and higher number for "water adjusted" target heart rates (e.g., 132 - 17 = 115 and 171 - 17 = 154).

for only six seconds and multiplying by 10 (just add a zero). If you are working aerobically this six-second numeral will be within your THRZ.

Check your pulse about five minutes into training and again when you're almost finished. You will want your heart rate to be between your target high and low for a minimum of 20 minutes.

Table 3.2
Six-Second Hydro-Heart Rate Chart

Age	Maximum heart rate	60% intensity heart rate	75% intensity heart rate	85% intensity heart rate
20-29	190-200	12	15	17
30-39	180-190	11	14	16
40-49	170-180	11	14	15
50-59	160-170	10	13	15
60-69	150-160	10	12	14
70 and up	150	9	11	13

This table should be used only as a guideline to average heart rates. The estimated maximum heart rates are appropriate. Consult your doctor for personal THR information.

Another quick method to monitor your intensity, called "Rating of Perceived Exertion" (RPE), asks you to listen to your body. Do you feel like you are exercising yet? Are you slightly winded or very winded? Now, equate how you feel you are working to a numeral on the scale of 0 to 10, with the number 10 being very, very hard, and 0 being not at all (see table 3.3). Perceived exertion is particularly useful if you have trouble counting the beats of your heart due to the wave action of the water or other distractions. It actually can be a more accurate measure of intensity than THR for some people, because it is much quicker.

Table 3.3
Borg's CR-10 Scale*

0	Nothing at all
0.5	Extremely weak (just noticeable)
1	Very weak
2	Weak (light)
3	Moderate
4	
5	Strong (heavy)
6	
7	Very strong
8	
9	
10	Extremely strong (almost max)
•	Maximal

*Category (C) scale with ratio (R) properties.

Reprinted by permission, from G. Borg, 1982, A Category scale with ratio properties for intermodal and interindividual comparisons. In *Psychophysical judgment and the process of perception*, edited by H. G. Geissler and P. Petzold (Berlin: VEB Deutscher verlag der Wissenschaften), 25-34.

Interpreting Your Scores

Your first set of test results establishes a base score for you to measure changes as they occur. Change is a fact of life and, with sound fitness goals, you will be pleased with the changes happening in your life. For some, just holding onto the status quo means success. National standards are mentioned to help you obtain and maintain recognized healthy levels in cardiovascular fitness and body composition. Don't let these standards cause you to compete with the population of the whole nation. Compete with yourself, trying to be just a little better than you were last month or last year at this time.

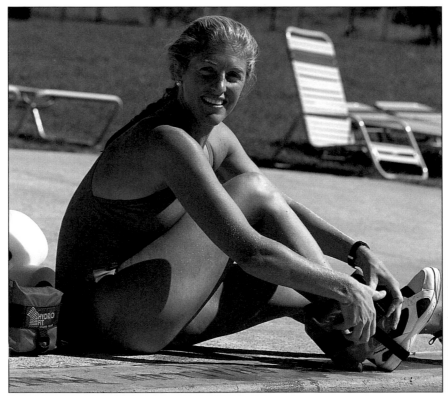

©F-Stock/ Gretchen Palmer

People of all fitness levels enjoy aquatic exercise.

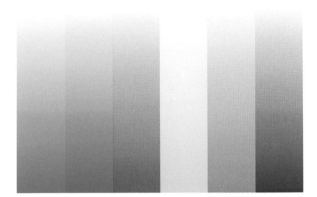

Aquatics the Right Way

Water is very polite. If you fall, it's there to catch you. It never pushes you harder than you push it, and it constantly nudges you gently toward the surface and into motion. Some people try water fitness once and go home with the resolve that it was too easy or too hard for them. How many activities exist that you can try once and perform well? The more hours you accumulate in the water, the better you'll be able to harness its power and understand how to make it work. In this chapter, the mechanics of each movement will be described. The terms I use will bring to mind familiar movements on land, but the moves will not necessarily feel the same or target the same muscles. Keep an open mind, listen to your body, and learn the secrets of the water.

Starting Out on the Right Foot

Watch people as they enter the water. A few plunge in with no hesitation; most raise their shoulders up to their ears and try to keep their elbows dry while inching in on tiptoe. The safest way to enter a pool is to back down the ladder or ease yourself in at an appropriate depth.

Acclimate your body to the water temperature, pressure, and buoyancy; adjust your breathing rate, maintain a relaxed neck and shoulders, and use the full foot as you move.

Good body alignment is almost an exercise in itself. It all begins at the feet. When you move slowly forward or sideways through the water, each foot should roll through its entirety—heel, ball, toe. At a fast pace (in place or moving any direction) when the body is ahead of the foot, the foot roll is reversed—toe, ball, heel. The heel must touch down with every step you take. Remember to keep the toes pointing in the same direction as the knee. Deep-water footwork alternates pointed and flexed positions, to contrast the muscles used.

Standing tall improves strength in the abdominal muscles and back muscles. Balance between these two muscle groups keeps the buttocks tucked in and the ribs lifted which keeps the shoulders relaxed and down, which in turn keeps the neck tall and tension-free. When the neck is where it's supposed to be, the chin is tucked in and centered over the chest, a more natural position than it sounds, and more comfortable than slouching. Seemingly small details like slouching or sloppy strokes actually cause you to feel tired, and you won't reach as effectively the muscles you intend to work.

Learn to avoid two common errors during water exercises: poor posture and poor breathing. In deep water, most people naturally begin swimming and lose control of good vertical posture, partly because there is less for the feet to push against. Because body fat floats, the front or back of your body may be pulled more than the other side to the surface, and the abdominal muscle group receives a great workout without consciously trying. Be aware of your personal needs. Keep the abdominals tight and your spine vertical. Use buoyant equipment to balance your body as comfortably and vertically as possible.

Breathe deeply and evenly during all activity—oxygen is an essential ingredient that fuels your muscles, and your oxygen consumption is used to measure the number of calories burned during activity. Deep breathing is harder in the water than on land, due to the weight of the water on the torso, so with each breath the diaphragm and lungs are getting stronger, reacting to the added resistance of the water. Exhale on the exertion and inhale on the recovery. On land or in water, adults commonly breathe with only one-third the capacity of their lungs. People who smoke or have limiting lung conditions can spend time systematically improving their lung capacity with bobbing and deep breathing in the water.

If you find it tough to remember all of a workout once you're in the pool, you might try one of the following memory aids:

- Practice poolside in front of a mirror.
- Mount notes on two kickboards leaning back to back or on a "wet floor" sign.
- Write aerobic combinations onto flashcards and laminate. Place them on the pool deck for quick reference or float them on kickboards.
- Copy the page you plan to use and place it in a plastic bag to post poolside.
- Work out with a friend and take turns calling out instructions.
- Use the "add-on" technique: Memorize exercises A and B. Repeat them until you're comfortable; then *add-on* exercise C. When you're comfortable with those three, add on the next and so on.

The most important thing to remember is to have fun and do what you do well and with full concentration. If you forget something, just move on. After one or two sessions, most everyone gets into a groove and does fine.

Basic Stances

Most water exercises begin in one of the following basic stances:

- **Basic**—stand with feet facing forward, shoulder-width apart, and knees relaxed. Hold the chest forward and press the shoulders down and back. Keep the abdominals tight. The arms should be relaxed at your side, with the thumbs toward the front.
- **Lunge**—place either foot one stride in front of the other. Keep both knees soft and point toes straight ahead. The front knee should not extend past the toes. The arm opposite the front foot is also forward. This very stable position provides great protection for your back as you do isolated upper-body work.
- **Astride**—extend each foot out to the side an equal distance from the center. The feet are usually most comfortable at a 45-degree angle.
- **Supine**—the front of the body lies facing up on the surface of the water. You may assume this stance while floating, holding the wall, or using flotation equipment.
- **Prone**—the front of the body lies facing down on the surface of the water. You may assume this position while floating, holding onto the wall, or using flotation equipment.

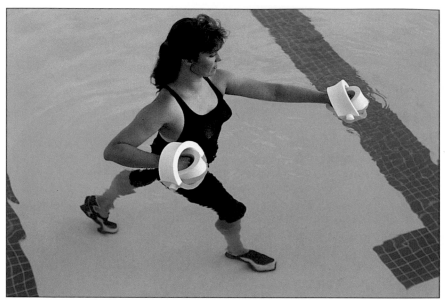

Lunge position

The Moves

The exercises described here start with the most basic, then move from less intense to more intense. You can also vary the intensity by how much you like an exercise, and your enthusiasm for the water. Arm movements are listed first. Leg movements are generally paired with a natural and complementary arm movement. Feel free to mix and match any combination that feels best to you. Remember, this is a water workout, so your arms should be in the water, using its resistance. Use your arms to help you change directions, to balance, or to increase the intensity of the exercise. The more muscles you move, the more aerobic the workout will be.

Customizing Your Workout

To add variety and vary the intensity of your workout, every shallow-water exercise can be performed in three different ways: suspended, neutral, and rebound:

- **Suspended**—lower your body neck-deep in the water. Although the floor is right there, your toes never touch the bottom. Your hands scull a small forward-and-backward figure-eight motion to keep you afloat. In this position, you can perform a variety of moves. Your shoulders have no vertical movement. This variation is

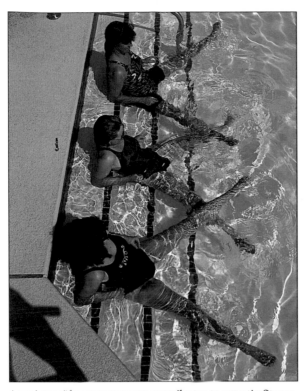

A variety of leg movements contributes to aquatic fitness.

challenging indeed, and an excellent change for short spurts, to rev things up.

• **Neutral**—standing chest-deep in the water, simply touch the bottom with your feet with each move. Support the majority of your weight with the water. Movement in any direction utilizes the weight and resistance of the water. The shoulders have minimal vertical movement.

• **Rebound**—push off the bottom of the pool from one or both feet. Lower the shoulders to near or below the water surface and then propel explosively skyward. Rebound is springy, splashy, bouncy. Breathe deeply, act like a child again, and make sure you are having fun.

While rebounding, your muscles rest for a few seconds as you wait for gravity to do its job. These exercises are referred to as "buoyancy-assisted moves." You are really only working half the time. The more of a "floater" you are, the more buoyant time you will have. You can make good use of this recovery time and make things more intense by pulling and pushing muscles purposefully in each direction before you land. Check the suggested variation for jumping jacks and cross-country ski for examples of maximizing rebound moves. Otherwise, keep jumping and enjoy the ride!

Here are ten ways to vary the workout intensity of your water exercises:

• Speed	• Leverage	• Rebound variation
• Rhythm	• Pattern	• Equipment
• Effort	• Suspended variation	
• Direction	• Neutral variation	

The Upper Body

The entire torso musculature works as a stabilizer during all upper-body work. Abdominal muscles work especially hard any time you pull down with long-lever arms. When you focus on the upper body, keep your legs stable in the lunge, basic, or astride position to protect your back from overexertion. If the knees are relaxed, the back usually will be relaxed, too. Keep the shoulders down and relaxed. You may want to do one arm at a time. Try these exercises without equipment first.

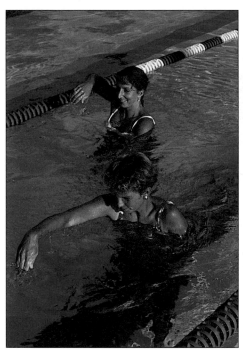

Fitness aquatics exercises the entire upper body.

Biceps/Triceps Curls

Keep the elbows stationary at your waist and keep the upper arm motionless. Pull the palms forward and upward toward the surface of the water, adjusting the speed so you feel the resistance of the water. Reverse the palms, facing them toward the floor, and press down and back with equal force until the arm is extended slightly behind the hips. You can work the same muscles with your arm held in different positions. Try your elbows elevated at your sides on the surface of the water. Your palms pull the water towards your chest and then push out.

Variation: Alternate arms.

Canoe Arms

Bring both hands forward about waist-high, palms down. Placing them together, forcefully draw both palms diagonally down and past your hip on one side (like a canoe paddle stroke). Return to the center quickly and repeat on the other side. You may be able to push forcefully enough to give your feet a lift off the bottom.

Big Claps/Scissors

Extend each arm out to the side, palms facing forward. Knees should be bent enough that the water is near your shoulders. Skimming straight arms along the surface of the water, pull both hands in front as if you wanted to clap. Reverse the palms and press back with equal speed and pressure to your starting position. Nice in a lunge position or while jogging backward.

Deep Pulls

With your legs in lunge position, pull both arms forward from your hips to the top of the water. Palms are to the front, scooping the water vigorously. Quickly reverse direction and force the water back with the palms as far as the arms will comfortably go. Try to develop a rhythm and maintain a full range of motion at the shoulder joint. Your body weight should stay centered and get an occasional lift as the arms push down.

Variations: Work double-time, with a smaller range of motion. Alternate arms in opposition to each other. Keeping the feet together, let your whole body be propelled forward and back as your arms push and pull.

Lateral Raises

With arms straight at your sides, simply lift the arms forcefully up and away from your body until they reach the surface of the water, then return with equal zeal to the starting position.

Variations: Turn the palms, increase speed, or add equipment to increase resistance.

Sideways Swings

With the elbows soft, swing the straight arms just in front of your hips and out to the side, first to the left and then to the right, both in unison. Turn the palms to maximize resistance.

Variations: Cup hands, slice, or add equipment.

Bow-and-Arrow Arms

This combination of moves uses virtually all the muscles in the upper chest. Begin with both arms extended, in front of your chest or over to one side, on the surface of the water. One arm bends at the elbow and retracts until the hand is near the shoulder, as if drawing the string on a bow. The arm then extends straight out to the side, still on the water's surface, and returns to the original position, pulling water the complete distance. The other arm stays put, awaiting its turn. Finish one set of 8 to 20 on one arm, then repeat on the other side.

Figure-Eights

With single arms to the side or both arms to the front moving in unison, use a fairly straight arm as you draw a figure-eight on its side. Move the hand in a diagonal manner until it can reach no further. Rhythmically and without stopping, curve down or up 12 inches so you can start another diagonal that, after curving again, has you back to where you started.

Power Arms

Bend elbows at 45-degree angles. With palms, push water to the front, slice the water, or relax and go along for the ride. The emphasis is on the elbows, which slide powerfully on a track equally far to the front and the back. Probably the most natural movement we use.

Funky Arms

Raise the arms forward to the surface of the water (about shoulder level). Press both palms to one side, circling in to the shoulders and forward again to where you started. There is some nice resistance while the arms are moving extended in a long lever. A great exercise paired with any sideways movements.

You can vary this list of favorite upper-body moves further with different hand positions. A small change from a slice to a fist can increase the intensity noticeably.

The Lower Body

The lower body is the focal point of most workouts, because that is where we have the majority of our muscle mass. There are only so many ways to move a muscle, but by changing combinations and patterns each workout can be very different.

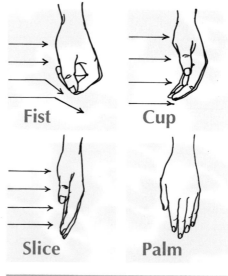

Fist   Cup

Slice   Palm

Figure 4.1   Hand positions change the intensity also.

Pedal

Stand tall, feet a few inches apart. Alternately roll up one heel and then the other. The balls of the feet should not leave the ground. At the same time, bring the straightened opposite arm forward, the palm pulling to the front as the arm moves backward, close to your side, facing the palm to the rear.

Variations: Work slowly, or pick up the pace. Add funky arms. Add triceps presses.

Water-Walk

Step forward as if walking on land. The heel strikes the bottom first and rolls smoothly forward through the length of the foot, to push off with the ball of the foot. The opposite arm moves forward with the leg that swings forward. There is no bounce to basic water-walking.

Variation: Be sure to include almost equal amounts of motion forward, backward, and sideways. Anything you can think of brings health gains.

Walking on Water

Stand on your left leg and lift the right leg to the surface of the water. Bring both arms forward, palms facing out on either side of the right ankle. As you leap forward, push the arms out and back, using them to propel and lift the body as if you could walk on the water. As the right leg lands on the floor the left leg rises to the surface and both arms slice forward, ready to propel you again. Raise the big toe out of the water (if it's comfortable) and leap as high as you can.

Two-Step

While walking, step forward two times, leading with the right leg and hip. Only shuffle the left foot up to the heel of the right leg to shift body weight. Let the hip follow the lead leg enough that your torso is almost turned sideways. Repeat, with the left leg leading. Pick up the pace once you get a rhythm established.

Variation: Try a backward two-step.

March/Jog

Alternately lift one knee, then the other, no more than hip-high. Pump the arms, slightly bent, forward and back, in opposition to the legs (as the right knee lifts forward the left arm is also forward). Marching always has one foot on the ground. Jogging is a little faster and involves some "air" time.

Variation: Kick heels up in back. Use longer arms, dragging the palms.

Bob

Begin in the basic stance and flex both knees to bring the chin to the surface of the water. Straighten the legs with an energetic push upward through the water and repeat, breathing deeply. Your arms should push down as your legs straighten, to help lift the body out of the water. If you're feeling more adventurous, go right under the water; exhale while you're under and inhale when you bob above the surface.

Variations: Make a quarter-turn each time you bob. Try a one-legged bob. Hold one leg to the side while bobbing.

Side Step/Gallop

Step out to the right side with the right leg and bring the left leg over to meet it. The shoulders and torso remain facing forward. Increase the speed to double-time and the side step takes on a bounce to become a gallop. Your body moves with the waves. In deep water the arms become more important if you really intend to move.

Variations: Countdowns of 8, then 6, then 4, then 2 are fun. Grapevine: Bring the left leg past the right ankle, alternately stepping in back and in front.

Double-Racquet Swing

A great water-walking step. Imagine you have a racquet in each hand. As you step forward with the left leg, swing the right arm forward from the side, fully extended and parallel to the floor, until it is midway in front of your torso. Step forward with the right leg and swing the left arm just the same, as if hitting a ball. Slow full range of motion makes this exercise a challenge.

Rocking-Horse

Standing in a lunge position, shift all your body weight forward onto the front foot. Place arms straight out front with palms on the surface of the water, and push both arms back and down. Shift your weight onto the back leg and pull both arms firmly forward. Complete one set of 10 to 20 with one leg leading, and then step forward to change legs and repeat another set.

Variations: Change the lead leg every fourth time by turning your torso before your weight shifts to the back leg. You will be facing the opposite direction, and what was the front leg is now the back! Double-time or double bounce. Move arms in opposition rather than together.

Tuck and Extend

Standing in a lunge position, draw the knee of the extended leg forward in front of the torso and quickly return it to the extended position. The elbows are also bent and move in opposition to the legs. Develop a strong rhythm as you pump out the set number on one leg, and then repeat on the other.

Jumping Jacks (the Aquatic Way)

Start with your feet together, arms straight to the sides on the surface of the water (you should look like a capital letter "T"). Jump up and move the legs sideways to a wide stance and pull the arms down to your sides as you land. Jump again and return to your starting "T" position. A bit of a coordination test for some people (but worth the extra effort), the arm and leg motions must *counteract* each other. This variation translates into fewer waves in the shallow water, and it is essential to keeping your head above water while in deep water.

Variations: Inside only—move the legs out and back in before your feet touch the ground. Straddle only—pull the legs to the center and back out before touching down. Alternately cross the arms in front and in back while jumping.

Giant Kick

Starting with the basic stance, kick one straight leg forward and up, no more than hip-high. Extend the opposite arm forward. Jump up and switch legs and arms. One leg will always be up. Repeat in a fluid, rhythmic motion, changing legs in midair.

Variations: Use small kicks, with a very straight leg, arms folded over the chest. Emphasize pulling down, faster or slower, diagonal kicks, lifting the leg slightly off center, or backward lifts. Be sure to keep your abdominals tight and chin slightly lowered, to protect your back.

Leg Swing

From the basic stance, lift one leg forward as the opposite arm swings forward. Bend the weight-supporting leg slightly and push off, for a small bounce as the lifted leg swings back. Pay attention to posture and keep the abdominals tight. The arms should pump freely in opposition to the legs. Repeat many times on one leg and change sides. Leg swings look like a simple exercise but can be very intense.

Variations: Swing with a bent knee. Count down: 16, 8, 4, 2, and 1!

Cross-Country Ski

Begin in the lunge position with the hands cupped for extra drag. One palm is always facing forward as the arm swings by your side to the front, while the other is facing back, arm swinging to the back. Jump up and bring the back leg to the front, landing with the knee bent and the rear leg straight. Change the arms simultaneously.

Variations: Switch legs in midair before your feet touch down. Try triceps extensions or biceps curls. Move forward through the water.

The Total-Body Twist

Twisting begins in the basic stance. Your body must move as one unit. Shoulders, hips, and knees move together, with the spine straight. The arms are extended at the surface of the water, far to the side opposite where you are facing. Bend both knees slightly and propel yourself off the bottom. Use the strength of your arms, pushing to the other side, to turn the torso and have the feet, knees, and shoulders end up pointing to the left, then right. Repeat.

Variations: Use a smaller range of motion, faster. Try in the suspended mode.

Pendulum Kick

From a basic stance, raise one leg straightened to the side. Press both palms to the opposite side. Hop and swish the arms and legs from side to side like the pendulum of a clock. Pull down hard; the moving leg may even gently knock the stationary leg out from under you.

Variations: Count four and turn to the right. Continue until you have faced north, south, east, and west. Then turn to the left. Try double-time, smaller.

Slalom Downhill

From a basic stance, bring the feet closer together. Hands are slightly forward as if you were holding ski poles. Keep the abdominals tight! Push both arms down and to the right as both knees lift and the feet land slightly to the left. Lift knees again and land the feet and knees to the right while pushing both arms to the left. If you have never skied, this move will look as if both legs are jumping to the right of a line on the floor and then to the left. The shoulders face forward and stay centered over the line.

Variations: Try the suspended mode. Jump over the imaginary line facing forward. Push legs forward, then back. The arms move in the opposite direction. Try doubles: two touch-downs on each side.

Tires/Cowboy Jog

Like the drill done during football practice, imagine you are running through two parallel rows of tires. Jogging in place keep the legs out wide and knees high. One leg is up while your weight is on the other.

Variations: Move forward, sideways, back, or in a circle.

Double Knee Tuck

Arms begin extended to the sides or front of the torso. Exhale and lift both knees toward the chest, keeping the abdominals tight. As the knees lift, push down with the arms, helping to keep you afloat. Return the feet to the floor and arms to the side.

Hamstring Curl

Bend at the knee to raise one heel up in back. Return it to the floor and repeat on the other side. The knee should stay pointed toward the floor or slightly back to engage the back of the thigh.

Variation: Two curls on one side before changing legs.

Lunge

Begin in the basic stance. Take an exaggerated step forward with the right leg, leaving the left foot in place. Press both arms back, helping to propel you forward as you step. The bent knee will be over the ankle. Reverse the arms, pulling forward, and push off with the front leg, returning to the center. Repeat on the other leg. Lunging to the side involves simply turning the torso and the right leg to the right as you extend the leg. It is a little more demanding because you move more water.

Variations: Add a bounce and you can bound forward, alternating legs and using opposite arms swinging at the sides. Fun combined with any arm action.

Power Squat

In the basic stance, press the buttocks down and back as if sitting in a chair. Pay attention to your knees—they stay centered over the foot and do not bend much. Squeeze the gluteals tight and return to basic stance. Try stepping out to your side as you squat. Let the torso move slightly to that side but still facing forward. Alternate left and center, right and center, for a powerful aerobic move.

Variations: Squat and lift in a step to the side, raising the free leg straight up and to the side. Repeat, stepping to the other side. The lower the gluteals move or the farther you step away when you step, the more water the straight leg potentially can lift. Squats are great when combined with a squat knee lift, or squat hamstring curl. Numerous arm exercises work well with squats.

Deep-Water Training

Deep-water training is the ultimate calorie burner, a pure no-impact workout. No impact means no pain and even less chance of injury, with more of your body under water. Deep water gives you total freedom to maximize your flexibility. A runner takes fewer steps while running in water yet each leg meets with increased resistance. Performing in water deeper than your height, you should be supported by a flotation device just buoyant enough to keep your chin at water level. Flotation equipment has little effect on intensity compared to its profound effect on comfort and technique. You don't need to know how to swim to get the benefits of deep-water training. Having the courage to embark on a deep-water training program opens a whole new world for many people. Be sure that there is a trained lifeguard on deck, and that you are secure with your flotation.

Deep water accommodates all fitness levels. Different movements create different workloads. Generally speaking, if you move with similar speed as in shallow water, deep water will be more intense, because you encounter more resistance and engage a greater muscle mass.

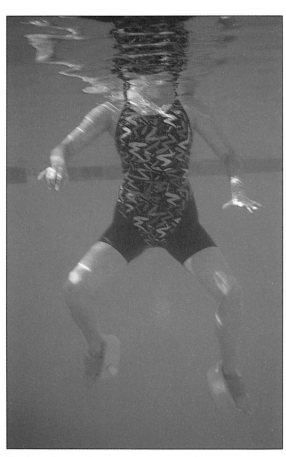

Deep water posture

Tips for Success in the Deep

Pushing and pulling your arms and legs through the water may not get you anywhere. If that's the case, congratulations! You are working the muscles in balance. One motion should counteract the other, leaving you in the same place. A knee or elbow brought so high in front should be brought so high in back. Focus on equal movement of the opposing muscles. Your workout is actually intensified when you use a tether to secure yourself in one place while you swim or run. Without the assistance of a current, working in place can increase the calories burned.

Locomotion comes with a planned change in hand position. Imagine your fingers are like the rudder of a boat. Turn your rudder out, away from the body, to move backward. Turn your rudder in to move forward. Everything else stays the same.

Posture is really important in deep water because you may be in that same position for a long time. Remember: chin pulled in, shoulders down and back, abdominals tight. When vertical, keep the spine fairly straight with no more than a 5-percent lean forward.

Deep-Water Running/Basic Jog

Use a similar motion as you would running on land. One knee lifts forward no more than hip-high, while the arm of that same side pulls back, with the elbow leading. The opposing leg raises to the back, also in a slightly bent position. Pull both knees down firmly, with the legs almost straightening as they pass directly underneath your torso. Imagine yourself pushing off the pavement. Each leg follows through a full range of motion, raising in the front and extending fully in the back. Your hands should be relaxed, the wrist in line with the forearm, which moves forward and back as if on a track very close to the rib cage. Unlike swimming, there is no circular motion. Stay vertical to maximize resistance and never allow the torso to lean too far forward or too far back. A 5-percent lean is most common.

Gallop

Take off in the basic run and add an exaggerated knee bend in both legs. Push down forcefully, imagining you can step right onto the water and lift yourself a foot or two higher. Move arms and legs twice as fast as in basic. The elbows come an inch or so away from your body for added lift as they pump back and forth, giving a very bouncy motion. When done correctly, the shoulders will rise high out of the water with each forceful thrust of the legs.

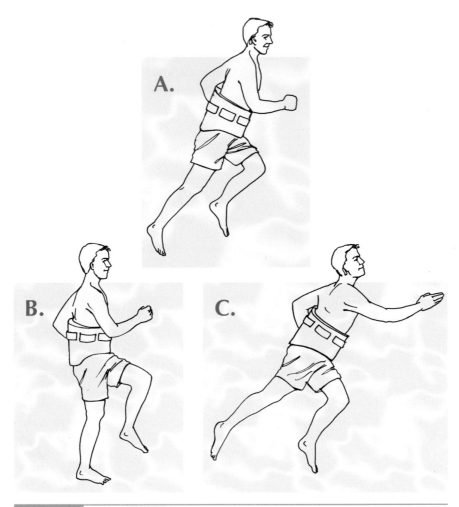

Figure 4.2 Deep Water Walking/Running: Lean slightly forward in the water as if you were running outdoors (see A.). B. and C. show two common, incorrect postures. Progress slowly through the water, or stay in place using the exact motion you would on dry land.

Pistons

Perform in place. From the basic run bring both knees forward and up high. Tighten the abdominals and alternate, quickly punching the feet down straight below you. Vary the foot position between toes pointed and foot flexed. The arms are moving in a much smaller range of motion and very fast. Pistons look a lot like a temper tantrum. Your shoulders should be shaking back and forth and making lots of waves.

Water Polo Goalie

Perform in place. From the basic run position take both knees forward and out wide to 45 degrees. This is the only exercise where your arms are not in opposition to your legs. Push the right arm and leg down through the water trying to lift the torso. Repeat with the left side. Pick up the pace. The shoulders should move quickly side to side in response to the leg movement, giving a lift to the whole body.

Vertical Flutter Kick in Place

Use a small, tight range of motion. With straight legs, and with your arms straight by your side, begin an alternating left, right flutter kick, pointing the toes for a set and then flexing the feet. The arms move opposite the legs, straight and tight. Focus your mind on the vertical lift. Feel your neck reach up to the sky.

Flicking

With the torso upright, sit in the water, knees flexed and the lower leg pointed down. Keep the thighs stationary and kick only the lower leg front and back, enough to propel you forward. Reverse the emphasis of the kick and move in reverse.

Abdominals

Abdominal muscles work nonstop as stabilizers during your entire deep-water workout. Include a few of these exercises after a workout, for extra credit. Aqua bars, Gyrojoggers, kickboards, or some other buoyant device held in each hand will give you added control with these exercises. They also work great with bare hands moving in a sculling motion to keep you stable.

Tucks. Lean slightly on your back, with arms out to the side for balance, legs together and extended. Tuck both knees to your chest as your arms pull in the direction of your feet. Contract the abdominal muscles. Return to the starting position and repeat. These moves can be done vertically, horizontally, or anywhere in between.

Diagonal Extensions. Lean slightly on your back, with arms extended out to the side for balance, legs together and straight. Tuck both knees to your chest as your arms pull toward the direction of your feet. Contract the abdominals. Turn the hips slightly to face one side and extend the legs to that side about 45 degrees from the starting position. Tuck the knees to the center, open the arms out to the side, then extend to the opposite side. This combination counts as one repetition. Not recommended for those with low back problems.

Twists. Extend the arms out to the side for balance. Draw the straight legs forward to a 90-degree position as if you were sitting on the floor. Pull down gently, about 1 inch, on the flotation in one hand. Tightening the abdominals, exhale and slowly let the legs rotate until they are under one hand. Inhale and repeat the process, slowly moving the legs over to the other hand. It will look like they are sliding on a horizontal piece of glass.

Pendulums. Extend the arms out to the side for balance, the legs straight down, keeping the spine straight. Pull down gently, about 1 inch, on the flotation in one hand. Tightening the abdominals, exhale slowly and let both legs raise together straight to the side under the extended arm. Pull down on the other arm; the legs will slowly raise to that side, swinging like the pendulum of a clock.

Horizontal Moves

When you first start a swimming program it is really important to master the basics first. Most people start with freestyle or the crawl. When you are really comfortable with the stroke, breathing rhythm, sharing lanes, and so on, then you should add to your repertoire of strokes.

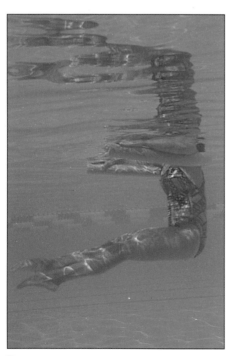

Deep water moves

Basic Swim Strokes

Typically you think swimming strokes involve the whole body, but when you talk about strengthening muscles, swim strokes are just as effective when isolated into upper-body and lower-body motions. Take that one step further and use only one arm or leg, to perform form, to simplify, or to intensify or correct an imbalance. Upcoming workouts will use swimstrokes in both vertical and horizontal positions. Before you can truly swim you need to be able to float and breathe rhythmically under the water. If you already swim well, these next few pages can freshen your skills.

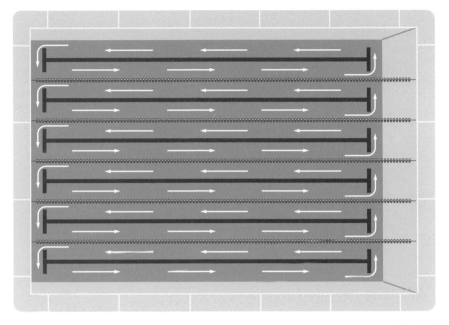

Figure 4.3 Traffic Patterns: If three or more swimmers are sharing a lane, they should swim in a circle, passing opposing swimmers on the right, similar to driving a car. To pass a swimmer going in the same direction, tap the slower swimmer on the foot. When the slower swimmer gets to the end of the lane, she should hesitate, allowing the faster swimmer to pass. If two swimmers share a lane, each swimmer can stay on the same side of that lane throughout the period.

The Crawl

The crawl (or freestyle) is the stroke most often used for fitness swimming. It burns more calories than some of the other strokes yet is easy to rack up the yardage without too high a risk of overuse. Begin this stroke with your chest down in the water and arms extended in front of you. In the crawl, your arms give most of the thrust; the legs move mostly to stabilize the body and keep it flat atop the water. Start pulling with the arm opposite the side you breathe on. Your hand enters the water first, with the fingers relaxed and gently cupped. It should be a clean entry without a lot of splash. Elbows and wrists are always above the fingers. Press down until your hand is about 10 inches below the surface, then pull it back toward your thigh in a slight "S" motion. After the power part of the stroke, that one shoulder rolls slightly upwards so you can lift your hand from the water, reaching forward with the elbow bent 45 to 90 degrees, ready for the next stroke. As one arm is beneath the body the other arm is in the air, preparing to stroke again.

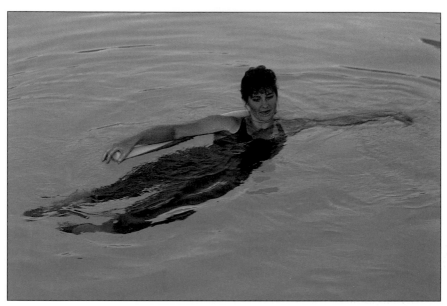

Even nonswimmers can enjoy deep-water exercise with proper flotation equipment.

Plan to turn your head to whichever side is more comfortable. Breathing on every second stroke of that one arm is ideal. Take as much air as possible while the shoulder is raised and the torso is rotated slightly. Full lungs help keep you buoyant and give the oxygen needed to supply the working muscles.

The kick starts at the hip and the power undulates down the leg, ending with a snap of the ankle. Toes are pointed (but relaxed) to be streamlined. The hip and thigh of one leg push down while the heel of the same leg is lifting up. The leg almost straightens momentarily with the snap of the ankle. Legs and feet should not break the surface of the water; the turbulence and drag slow you down.

Each up-and-down movement of one leg is counted as one beat. A good beat ratio is to kick each leg three times for the stroke of one arm. Some people do better with two or four beats to a cycle. Just do whatever works for you, and try to be consistent.

Backstroke

With your back on the water, begin this stroke with one arm entering the water above your head, little finger first. The elbow leads as the palm catches water and pushes down toward your feet 8 to 12 inches under the water's surface. This power phase ends when your arm is straight and your hand is near the back of the thigh. At this point the arm is ready to lift again, beginning with raising that shoulder. One arm recovers as the other arm pulls. Try to keep your head aligned with your spine and let the torso roll slightly as you lift the next arm.

The kick for the backstroke is the same as for the crawl: continuous undulating up-and-down motion of the leg originating at the hip. The ankle should be loose and should emphasize the alternating upward kick motion.

Breathing is easy, since your face is always out of the water. Relax, try to breathe deeply, and develop a rhythm.

Breaststroke

Unlike the first two strokes described, the breaststroke uses both sides of the body in the same way at the same time. Both arms pull while the legs recover; the legs kick while the arms recover, producing an alternate rhythmic lifting of first the upper body, then the lower body.

Begin with a forward glide, face down in the water. The palms should be six to eight inches below the surface of the water. With the palms leading, press the straight arms out toward the corners. From this position bend at the elbows and, as the palms catch the water, use the forearms to pull down and out, keeping the elbows higher than the hands. When the forearms reach a vertical position, rotate the palms in toward each other, ending the power phase of the arms. Pull in to the center, almost clapping your hands. Follow the direction of the finger tips, recovering up the length of the torso and straightening the arms ahead in a glide position.

Bend your hip and knee as if the heels were going to kick the buttocks. The knees are pointing to the floor and the heels stay in the water. Separate the knees and pull the heels in toward the center while extending the legs quickly to full length. Power comes from pushing the water with the insides of the legs and the soles of the feet.

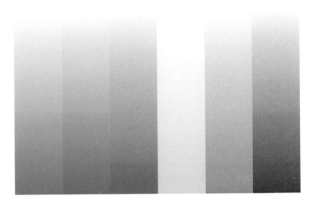

5

Warming Up and Cooling Down

Think of a dry piece of spaghetti. You can't bend it, stretch it, or pull on it—until it is warmed up. Raising the temperature and increasing blood flow to the muscles is what the warm-up is all about. After they are warmed up, muscles and joints will be looser, more flexible, and better prepared for action. Cool-down is the warm-up in reverse. If you stop cold while exercising full throttle or neglect to stretch, there can be complications and unnecessary pain. The following pages have ideas on how to warm up and cool down skillfully.

Warming Up

The first 5 to 10 minutes of each workout begins by using the large muscles of the body to get the blood pumping. The colder the water, the more vigorous or lengthy your warm-up should be. Warming up on deck does little to help, because once you hit the cooler water the muscles tighten back up again. Warm up in the medium where you will be working. Muscles, tendons, and joints will move more easily as their temperature increases. Warm muscles can also contract with greater force, through a wider range of motion, burning more calories. Warming up should bring your heart rate up to around 60 percent of maximum, or a fairly light perceived exertion of 4. Avoid using equipment during the warm-up unless it is for flotation in deep water.

Devote the last few minutes of your warm-up time to preparing specific smaller muscles that you plan to emphasize. Water-walks will focus on leg muscles. Prenatal and postnatal exercisers will concentrate on arm and postural muscles. Deep-water running requires a head-to-toe, total-body warm-up. Any exercise done at a slower pace and with a full range of motion can be considered a warm-up exercise. Not only will you be more comfortable when you gradually increase the demands on your body, but research has shown you will have improved performance and comfort, and reduce the chance of injury when you begin with a proper warm-up. Take 30 seconds right now to demonstrate to yourself these same research results.

To Warm Up or Not to Warm Up

Seated comfortably, lay either forearm on a tabletop or other flat surface. Be prepared to tap your pointer finger as fast as you can on that surface and count the number of taps. Set a timer for 15 seconds. GO! Write that number down. Now up on your feet for a nice gentle warm-up. March in place 20 times. Alternate clapping your hands in front of your body, then in back, for five repetitions. Circle your arms through the air as if you were swimming, 20 times. Do jumping jack arms 10 times. Reach your right arm to the sky and hold 10 seconds. Other side. March 10 times with a biceps curl. Play the piano in the air from left to right. Take three deep breaths and then go back to your seat with your forearm on a flat surface. Don't you feel better already? O.K. Exactly the same as before. Same arm, same finger, same length of time. Don't forget to count. GO!

Most people improve their counts up to 50 percent (if they can count that fast). What made the difference? Large, slow movements actually lubricate the joints, increased blood flow brings more oxygen to each and every cell, and a higher body temperature eases the ability of the muscles to be extended. Who would ever move without warming up, if they knew what you now know?

Warming up isn't just physical. It is also a mental wake-up call. Sometimes getting started is the hardest part. Clear your mind of outside thoughts. Use those first five to eight minutes to tune in to your body. Feel the power and potential that is there. Many people find their most creative ideas and solutions to problems during or soon after vigorous exercise.

Cooling Down

After completing the workout you will need to spend five to eight minutes in a cool-down phase. Like the warm-up, cool-down exercises can be similar to what you did in your workout but are performed more slowly and less intensely. Cool-downs will also be affected by the temperature of the water. Your large muscles should be kept moving slowly for five to eight minutes, incorporating the stretches listed on the next pages. Cooling down properly adds to your comfort after the workout, by giving your lungs, heart, and blood flow a chance to return to normal, easing muscle tension and reducing any chance of muscle soreness. Water workouts can even reduce soreness acquired in land-based activities. Stay in the water for cool-downs, letting the water continue to support you while your body gradually adjusts.

Stretching

For some people, stretching after exercise is about as entertaining as washing your hands or brushing your teeth after meals. You know you should, but there are more pressing things to do. Beginner or advanced, if you have them, stretch them! Your body is primed and most receptive

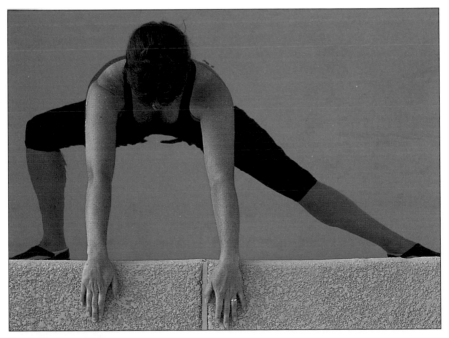

Stretching poolside

to stretches after everything is warm and well lubricated. Optional pre-stretches may be done after the warm-up but before the workout. Cool water reduces the benefits of stretching enough that you may want to keep the vigorous movement going and move straight into the workout. Stretching after the workout is referred to as post-stretch. Focus primarily on the muscles you contracted during the workout. Large muscle groups are done first, followed by medium-sized muscles. There are also benefits from stretching smaller areas like ankles and wrists, to increase joint mobility, range of motion, and comfort.

To stretch properly, simply elongate any warm muscle to a point of gentle tightness and hold for 20 to 30 seconds. There should be no bouncing and no pain. Every muscle has a small receptor that senses stretching of the muscle, a protective device that causes the muscle to clamp down and therefore not stretch too far. When you move into a stretch slowly and hold the stretch long enough, the receptor resets its acceptable length. You will feel the muscle relax and elongate. This relaxation feels wonderful and allows you to stretch further! Exhale deeply once you have established the stretching position to release more tension. If you feel the stretch in the muscle, good; if you feel tightening in a joint, you need to adjust your position. You can repeat the same stretch two or three times in succession. If stretching seems like forever because of cool water, try to keep other body parts moving while you stretch to keep warm. Long, slow stretching is the best way to stay supple and flexible.

Last of all, remember to breathe normally while stretching. Give those muscles all the oxygen they need. Listen to your body, ease into it, and make sure you really feel the stretching where you are trying to stretch. If you take the time to breathe and stretch correctly, you will reach deeper into the muscle to elongate, release tension, and increase circulation. With only minor adaptations, the same stretches work in deep and shallow water.

- Breathe deeply throughout the stretch.
- Generally do these stretches in the suggested order.
- Hold the stretch for at least 30 seconds or until you feel the muscle relaxing.
- No bouncing.
- Only gentle tightness.
- If it causes you pain, STOP and seek professional advice.

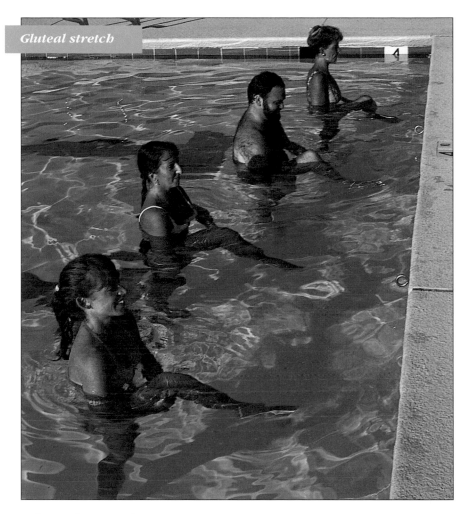

Gluteal stretch

Gluteal Stretch

Using both arms, grab your thigh just under the fold of your knee. Pull the thigh straight toward your chest and shoulders. Hold for 30 seconds. Use this same leg for the hamstring stretch.

Hamstring Stretch

Facing the pool wall, extend one leg forward and place the foot about hip-high. Bend at the waist slightly, keeping your spine straight. When gentle tightness is felt at the back of the leg, hold for 30 seconds or more. Use this same leg for the following quadriceps stretch.

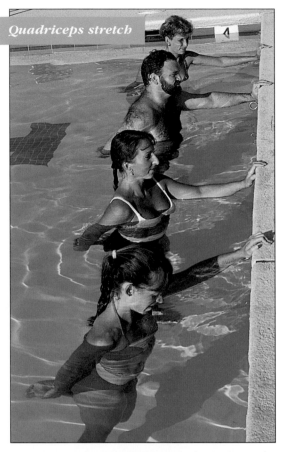

Quadriceps stretch

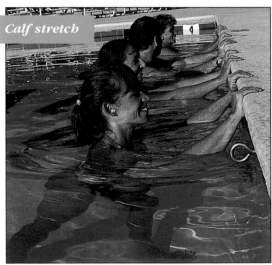

Calf stretch

Quadriceps Stretch

Standing tall, hold the pool wall or some flotation with one hand for stability. Bend the leg behind you, grasping the foot with the opposite hand. Begin with the knees close together and pointing down. Gently pull that leg back, being careful not to compress the knee. Hold for 30 seconds.

Calf Stretch

Holding something for balance, stand on one foot, knee and toes pointed straight ahead, knee bent slightly. Stretch your other leg straight back, rolling down (toe, ball, heel) to the floor. Hold for 30 seconds.

Repeat this sequence of four stretches on the other leg.

Anterior Lower Leg Stretch

Holding on, place all your weight on the forward leg. Let the top of the rear foot rest on the pool bottom. Gently push down and forward to feel the stretch. Hold. Repeat other side.

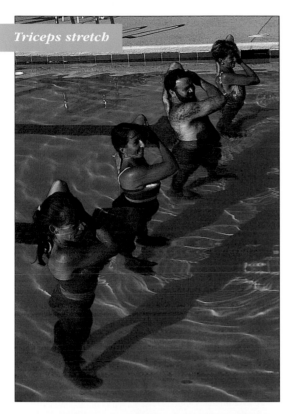

Triceps stretch

Triceps Stretch

Raise one arm to the sky; drop the hand behind your head so the elbow is pointing straight up. With your free arm gently press the upper arm backward, stretching the triceps. Hold for 30 seconds.

Posterior Shoulder Stretch

With both arms extended forward at shoulder level, pull above one elbow joint, bringing the arm in toward the shoulder. Feel the stretch in the posterior deltoids and upper back. Hold for 30 seconds and reverse sides.

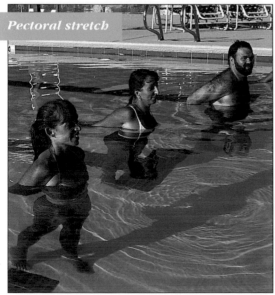

Pectoral stretch

Trapezius Stretch

With arms extended forward shoulder-high, grasp one wrist, palms facing out. Drop the chin to the chest and extend the arms a little farther forward. Round the shoulders slightly until you feel the stretch in the upper back. Hold for 30 seconds.

Pectoral Stretch

Extend arms behind the body. Grasp one wrist, pressing the shoulders

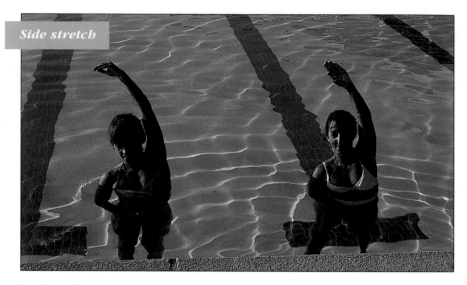

Side stretch

back and down. (Use a towel to connect your hands if needed.) Focus on opening up the rib cage. The wrists may be lifted or pressed down to increase the stretch. Hold 30 seconds and change hands.

Side Stretch

Stand with feet shoulder-width apart and knees relaxed. Extend either arm straight up toward the sky, keeping both heels on the ground. Lift the rib cage and feel the stretch from the hip, across the torso, and up the arm. Hold 30 seconds. Repeat on the other side.

Forward Neck Roll

Begin with the shoulders down and relaxed. Drop one ear towards the shoulder. Roll the chin forward and down slowly and up to the other shoulder. Feel the tension released in the back of the neck. If one place is especially tight, hold there until it relaxes. Continue to the other side, always keeping the head forward.

Ready for Aquatic Fitness!

You have estimated your current fitness level. You are familiar with the many ways to move your body in the water and you know the best way to start and end the workouts. Part II contains more ways to put aquatic workouts together in an enjoyable and healthy way. Let's take a look!

PART II

THE AQUATIC WORKOUT ZONES

The chapters in this book use six different color-coded workout zones, arranged according to duration and intensity. The brighter the color of the zone, the more intense the workouts. Each color is designed to keep you working within a set range of your individual maximum heart rate. For example, workouts in the Green zone will have you working at about 65 percent of your maximum; workouts in the Red zone will have you working at 85 percent to 90 percent.

Workouts progress in difficulty as you move within each zone. The first workouts will be the least demanding, whereas the last will be the most demanding. There is also a built-in progression of minutes spent in your training zone. Each workout has a specific training purpose, an arrangement that invites you to move back and forth from zone to zone as your training needs vary.

There is no easy way to measure the distance traveled in vertical deep-water workouts, or in some shallow-water workouts performed in place. The degree of difficulty in a workout is determined by how hard you are working, not how far you go. Intensity is correlated to how much water you move and how much muscle mass is in motion. Once you have learned to manipulate the water, then you can vary any workout to meet your training agenda, and you can exercise at the same time with others who are working at different intensities.

WORKOUT COLOR ZONES			
Zone (chapter)	Type of workout	RPE/ %MHR	Time
Green (6)	Low intensity, short duration	2–4/60–69	20–35 min
Blue (7)	Low intensity, long duration	2–4/60–69	25–55 min
Purple (8)	Moderate intensity, short duration	3–7/60–79	20–50 min
Yellow (9)	Moderate intensity, long duration	4–7/70–85	35–50 min
Orange (10)	High intensity, short duration	5–8/70–95	30–45min
Red (11)	High intensity, long duration	7–10/80–100	45–60min

Caloric Cost

The number of calories burned during each workout depends upon muscle mass, which is different for each person. Comparing calorie consumption, one mile of swimming roughly equals four miles of running on land. Predicting calories for swimming depends on speed, skill, and the stroke used. Interestingly, poor swimmers, because they are less efficient in their strokes, consume more calories than expert swimmers over the same distance. Poor swimmers typically take more strokes in a length than good swimmers and create a lot of turbulence for themselves with sloppy moves. This same turbulence is in part what maximizes the workload for vertical water exercise. Table II.1 gives an average of calories per minute burned during a variety of activities.

The ability to burn energy at the highest level depends upon your capacity to consume oxygen. The maximum rate of oxygen (VO_2) is the most accurate measure of energy output, because oxygen is required in converting fat to energy. An average active VO_2 for an untrained 160-

pound male is three liters per minute. For a female weighing 125 pounds, it is two liters per minute. That rate converts to about 14 to 15 calories per minute to maintain vigorous activity. The body's capacity to burn calories improves with regular participation in aerobic activities.

Table II.1
Aerobic exercises in water, wearing shoes (lower body, legs, hips)

Activity	VO_2 (ml•kg•min)	VO_2max	Heart rate (bpm)	%HRmax	kcal/min	kcal/hr
Running, forward/back	47	87%	168	82%	17	1020
Running in place	46	85%	164	80%	17	1020
(Compares with running 7 min/mile)					18	1080
Running, sideways	39	72%	162	79%	14	840
Running, boxed	39	72%	146	71%	14	840
Walking, power	44	81%	160	78%	14	840
(Compares with running 9 min/mile)					14	840
Treading/stride hops (front-back)	38	70%	143	70%	13	780
Leg thrusts, supine	43	79%	165	81%	15	900
Bobbing, waist-deep	42	77%	163	80%	15	900
Average*	42	78%	159	78%	15	892
(Compares with running 8 min/mile)					15	900

*Based on performing lower body *aerobic training* exercises, each an equal amount of time, in an aerobic circuit-training format.

Bob L. Beasley, Paul McGorry and Carlos Sanchez, Unpublished Data, 1986 PED 208 University of South Florida, Department of Physical Education

6

Green Zone

Workouts in the Green zone require the minimum physical output to improve or maintain your fitness level. In duration, they begin at less than 30 minutes and progress to 35 minutes. Working at about 60-percent intensity is a good pace for starting a new program. Highly trained sports enthusiasts will also find themselves in the Green zone for cross-training and an occasional no stress day. The slightly slower pace is a great opportunity to evaluate your form or rejuvenate sore muscles. Green zone workouts are especially effective for increasing flexibility and range of motion. Low-intensity, short-duration workouts also release stress, lower cholesterol levels, and improve muscle tone and circulation. Green zone workouts should be performed frequently during the week to achieve the desired benefits. Remember to listen to your body and work at the pace that's best for you.

Warm-Up A

Water walk three minutes, forward, backward, and sideways. Jumping jacks 10 times. Hip circles 10 times, each way.

Giant arm circles under the water, 10 forward, 10 back. Alternating side lunges 10 times, alternate heel touches to the front 8 times, heel touches to the side 8 times, toe touch in back 8 times. Repeat. Remember to move the arms in a similar action with the feet.

Warm-Up B

Water walk three minutes, forward, backward, and sideways. Four big inhales. Ten of everything. March in place. Deep pulls with slicing hands. Small bobs. Hands behind the back and rotate the trunk slowly with knees bent. Side lunges. Hook the thumbs together and with arms extended out front, draw a large figure-eight on its side.

Deep-Water Warm-Up

Two laps each of breaststroke, backstroke, and crawl. One minute easy basic run, in place. One minute cross-country ski. If you feel tightness or tension anywhere in the body, use the stretches beginning on page 57 as a pre-stretch after the warm-up.

WORKOUT 1

WATER-WALKING WORKOUT
TIME: 25 minutes

WARM-UP: A or B

WORKOUT

Location: Chest-deep water
Pace: Smooth and brisk
Effort: 2-3 RPE; 60-69% max HR
Activity:
Water-walk briskly 4 lengths forward, 4 backward, 8 sideways
Jog with crawl-stroke arms 2 lengths forward, 2 backward
Long strides and arms scooping the water 2 lengths
Cross-country ski 2 lengths
Jog 4 lengths sideways, working deep into the water with jumping jack arms
Step hop 2 lengths
Jumping jacks with alternate arm pulling backward 2 lengths
Total-body twist and push backward 2 lengths
Water-walk forward 4 lengths, backward 4 lengths, sideways 8 lengths

COOL DOWN AND STRETCH

COMMENTS

Don't turn around when stepping sideways. In cross-country ski, pull arms back forcefully to help you move.

2

BASIC WATER EXERCISES
TIME: 26 minutes

WARM-UP: A or B

WORKOUT

Location: Shallow water

Pace: Brisk

Effort: 2-3 RPE; 60-69% max HR

Activity:

10 bobs each, north, south, east, west

10 jumping jacks each, 4 directions

20 double knee tucks and triceps presses

30 cowboy jogs, elbows just above water

30 power jogs

For 4 sets: cross-country ski 15x in all directions; 10 rocking-horses w/right leg, 10 w/left

For 4 sets: 60 side lunges w/double-handed punch alternating sides; 60 hamstring curls w/bow-and-arrow arms alternating sides; 8 total-body twists w/legs together, 8 w/legs apart

60 kicks front while clapping under knee alternating sides

For 4 sets: side step 4x right, 4x left, scooping water with arms

Step hop in place 30x each direction

80 backward leg presses, alternating legs

Repeat entire workout

COOL DOWN AND STRETCH

COMMENTS

Refer to different hand positions (Figure 4.1, page 38) to vary the intensity of the workout. Be sure to keep your back straight.

JUMP AND SHOUT
TIME: 30 minutes

WARM-UP: A or B

3

WORKOUT

Location: Shallow water

Pace: Lively

Effort: 2-3 RPE; 60-69% max HR

Activity:

For 3 reps: easy march in place with 8 punches each—up, down, front, sides

30 knee lifts one side, 30 other side

20 jogs with heels up in back

30 bobs

For 4 reps: 8 total-body twist w/legs together, 8 apart

30 low straight leg kicks

For 10 counts, low kicks, legs in back, crawl-stroke arms moving forward

Reverse arms, take legs to the front

Kick back to where you started

For 3 reps: side step and scoop water with both arms 8 to the right, 8 left

30 bobs

30 cross-country ski

For 4 reps: 8 giant strides forward with breaststroke arms, 8 backward

30 pendulum kicks

Repeat entire workout

COOL DOWN AND STRETCH

WORKOUT 4

4

COMBINATIONS
TIME: 35 minutes

WARM-UP: A or B

WORKOUT

Location: Shallow water
Pace: Energetic
Effort: 3-4 RPE; 60-69% max HR
Activity:

60 steps marching in place

For 4 reps: giant strides with breaststroke arms, 8 backward, 8 forward

For 4 reps: 8 steps marching in place; 8 giant strides forward; 8 steps marching in place; 8 giant strides back

30 cross-country ski

For 4 reps: 4 side steps right, 4 left

For 4 reps: 8 cross-country ski, 4 steps right; 8 cross-country ski, 4 steps left

For 4 reps: jog in place and do 8 arm punches front, 8 sideways, 8 down, 8 up

30 bobs

For 4 reps: jog while punching 8x each direction, then 8 bobs

40 alternate hamstring curls

30 pendulum kicks

For 8 reps: 4 hamstring curls, 4 pendulum kicks

20 double knee tucks

For 4 sets: 20 total-body twist with wide stands; 4 knee tucks; 4 wide twists

Repeat entire workout

COOL DOWN AND STRETCH

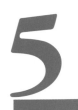

WAIST WORK

TIME: 30 minutes

WARM-UP: A or B

WORKOUT

Location: Shallow water
Pace: Energetic
Effort: 3-4 RPE; 60-69% max HR
Activity:

30 bobs, arms above head, pulling down as you jump up

30 total-body twists

40 side lunges alternating right, left

Jog forward with giant-butterfly arms for 1 lap

Jog backward with elementary backstroke for 1 lap

For 4 reps: side step 4 right, 4 left

30 cross-country ski

For 4 reps: 4 side steps right; 4 cross-country ski; 4 side steps left; 4 cross-country ski

60 bobs

30 slaloms

60 jogs

30 total-body twists

For 4 reps: 4 slaloms, 4 jogs, 4 twists

60 bobs

Repeat entire workout

COOL DOWN AND STRETCH

WORKOUT 6

6

LUCKY 32

TIME: 32 minutes

WARM-UP: A or B

WORKOUT

Location: Shallow water
Pace: Rebound
Effort: 3-4 RPE; 60-69% max HR
Activity:

Water jog for 3 minutes
Straight leg swing, 32 each leg
Rocking-horse, 32 each leg
32 giant kicks
32 cross-country ski
32 slaloms
32 slow jogs
32 quick jogs

Alternate fast and slow jogging for 64 steps
32 jumping jacks
32 tuck and lunge each side
32 bobs all 4 directions
32 giant kicks to corners
32 deep pulls

Repeat entire workout

COOL DOWN AND STRETCH

COMMENTS

Why "Lucky 32?" Physiologists report improvements in muscle tone occur with as few as 32 repetitions of any exercise.

BUTT BURNER
TIME: 30 minutes

WARM-UP: A or B

7

WORKOUT

Location: Shallow water
Pace: Lively
Effort: 2-3 RPE; 60-69% max HR
Activity:

Begin face up, holding onto wall or with kickboards under each arm

30 easy flutter kicks

Roll over, 30 easy flutter kicks

60 jumping jacks

40 giant kicks

Jog moderately hard 40 steps

40 cross-country ski

30 quick flutter kicks face up, 30 face down

45 pendulum kicks

60 bobs

30 single leg swings each side

30 slaloms

30 knee tuck lunges each leg

30 flutter kicks, relaxed but firm, face up, 30 face down

30 rocking-horses each leg

30 small forward kicks while pulling down

15 giant kicks

For 8 reps: 4 small kicks, then 2 giant kicks

Repeat entire workout

COOL DOWN AND STRETCH

COMMENTS

For a portion of this workout you will need to be near a wall or have a flotation device under each arm. Aqua bars or Gyrojoggers in each hand make the transition from vertical to horizontal exercise very smooth.

WORKOUT 8

CONDITIONING SPORT CIRCUIT
TIME: 21 minutes

WARM-UP: A or B

WORKOUT

Location: Shallow water
Pace: Brisk
Effort: 3-4 RPE; 60-69% max HR
Activity:

Station 1: 30 jumping jacks, 15 jumping jacks arms in front, 15 back

Station 2: 15 bobs, 15 butterfly arms

Station 3: 40 total-body twists, 40 canoe arms each side

Station 4: jog through tires 40x, 20 racquet swings, alternating sides

Station 5: 40 backward leg lifts, 40 power punches

Station 6: 30 hamstring curls, 30 big claps

Station 7: 60 jogs, 30 backstroke arms

Station 8: 40 rocking-horses each leg, 30 deep pulls

Station 9: 20 bobs forward, 20 back, 30 butterfly arms each direction

COOL DOWN AND STRETCH

COMMENTS

For this workout, isolate the lower body first, then the upper body. Keep knees bent to protect back and arms under water, which maximizes resistance.

HALF AND HALF
TIME: Variable

WARM-UP: A or B

WORKOUT

Location: Shallow water
Pace: Mark your times for future comparison
Effort: 3-4 RPE; 60-69% max HR
Activity:

1 length crawl stroke

35 bobs

1 length backstroke

40 jumping jacks

1 length breaststroke

40 pendulums

1 length pull only w/flotation between ankles

60 quick jogs

2 lengths your choice

60 cross-country ski

1 length kick only w/flotation between hands

40 butterfly arms in place

Repeat entire workout

COOL DOWN AND STRETCH

COMMENTS

If you have always wanted to swim lengths, this is the workout to get you started. Swimming requires endurance built up over time. Each swimming length ends with a set of vertical exercises that keeps the heart working but gives you time to breathe deeply before going on to the next length. You will need one flotation device to hold between your legs or hands for pull only and kick only.

WORKOUT 10

10

EASY SWIM
TIME: 25 minutes

WARM-UP: A or B

WORKOUT

Location: Shallow water
Pace: 25-35 seconds to cover 25 yards
Effort: 3-4 RPE; 60-69% max HR
Activity:
50 yards freestyle easy
50 yards pull only easy
50 yards kick only easy
50 yards backstroke
4 x 50 yards freestyle for 30 seconds each
100 yards backstroke

COOL DOWN AND STRETCH

COMMENTS

You may rest longer at the end of a length if needed. The important thing is to finish the workout.

7

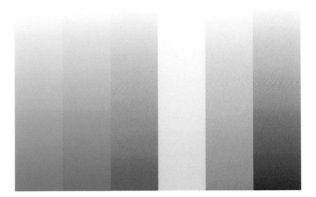

Blue Zone

The next 10 Blue workouts are still within the easy range of your heart rate or perceived exertion level. The moves are the same but the longer duration in your target zone challenges your endurance. Many athletes like to use the blue zone as a cool-down after land activities.

1

WATER-WALKING WORKOUT
TIME: 45 minutes

WARM-UP: A or B

WORKOUT

Location: Shallow water

Pace: Powerful

Effort: 3-4 RPE; 60-69% max HR

Activity: (All numbers are number of lengths.)

4 long, slow walk alternating forward, backward

4 sideways, stepping together

2 backward w/backstroke arms

1 forward total-body twist, 1 backward

2 power walking

2 scoop and jump forward, 2 backward

4 alternating two-step

2 jogging w/breaststroke arms

2 power walking

2 racquet step

(Right leg steps forward while left arm swings. Alternate sides.)

1 jumping jack facing forward, 1 backward

2 power walking

2 jogging sideways

2 double knee tucks moving backward

2 power walking

2 hurdle jumps

2 jogging w/ power arms

4 giant strides

2 power stride w/straight legs and arms

2 hamstring curls

2 fast jog, arms dragging behind

4 walking w/power arms, alternating forward, backward

COOL DOWN AND STRETCH

COMMENTS

Keep arms under water as much as possible. Take a minute to review the list of 10 ways to increase intensity. If you are working in a smaller area, give yourself 25-30 steps of each exercise to equal one length.

WORKOUT 2

WATER EXERCISE
TIME: 45 minutes

2

WARM-UP: A or B

WORKOUT

Location: Shallow water

Pace: Powerful

Effort: 3-4 RPE; 60-69% max HR

Activity:

For 4 sets: 20 marches, 20 cross-country ski, 20 bobs in all directions, 20 pendulum swings

50 rocking-horse on right leg

For 4 sets: 4 giant kicks, 4 jogs, 4 leg lifts in back, 4 hamstring curls

50 rocking-horse on left leg

For 4 sets: 8 jumping jacks, 4 twists left, 8 diagonal kicks, 4 twists right

50 fast jogs

For 4 sets: 4 forward lunges w/biceps curls

4 power squats to the sides w/bow-and-arrow arms

4 hamstring curls w/triceps press

2 jumps forward, 2 back

50 moderate jogs

COOL DOWN AND STRETCH

COMMENTS

Get that water surging and chopping all around you. Test your memory and, when you're done, repeat each set one more time.

WORKOUT 3

3

TONE AND TIGHTEN
TIME: 45-55 minutes

WARM-UP: A or B

WORKOUT

Location: Shallow water
Pace: Powerful
Effort: 2-3 RPE; 60-69% max HR
Activity:

16 power squats each side

8 jogs forward, 8 backward

For 4 reps: 4 jogs forward; squat right, then left; 4 jogs backward; squat right, then left

30 single leg swings each leg, w/opposite arm forward

30 total-body twists w/legs together, 30 w/legs apart

30 rocking-horses each side

45 cross-country ski

20 tuck and extends each side

45 double knee tucks

45 jogs through tires

25 hamstring curls each side

45 jumping jacks

25 diagonal kicks each side

60 hard jogs

40 pendulums

20 back leg lifts each leg

60 bobs

Repeat entire workout

Try for a third time!

COOL DOWN AND STRETCH

COMMENTS

All the moves in this workout focus on total body toning. Keep arms pumping forcefully in opposition to leg motion.

WORKOUT 4

ALL-AMERICAN
TIME: 45-50 minutes

4

WARM-UP: A or B

WORKOUT

Location: Shallow water
Pace: First time neutral; rebound the second
Effort: 3-4 RPE; 60-69% max HR
Activity:

Water-walk 4 minutes briskly
45 bobs
45 pendulum kicks
30 double knee tucks
45 cross-country ski
30 moguls
60 jogs through tires
30 hamstring curls
30 giant kicks
Side step 2 laps or step 8 right
    then 8 left for 4 reps
45 total-body twists
45 rocking-horses each leg

For 1 minute or one length each side, flutter kick on all 4 sides using a kickboard or the wall to support upper body
60 jogs in place
45 jumping jacks, crossing alternate arms in front and back
60 relaxed bobs

Repeat entire workout as high as you can in rebound mode

COOL DOWN AND STRETCH

COMMENTS

Focus on using the full range of motion, keeping the moves fairly neutral the first time through. This is a long, slow, fat-burning workout that includes a little bit of everything.

WORKOUT 5

5

BEST OF BOTH WORLDS
TIME: 45-50 minutes

WARM-UP: A or B

WORKOUT

Location: Shallow water
Pace: Energetic
Effort: 3-4 RPE; 60-69% max HR
Activity:

45 bobs

For 4 sets: 45 jogs, 45 pendulum kicks, 45 total-body twists

Jog in a box: 4 jogs forward, then make 1/4 turn; 4 jogs, and turn again, etc

Complete the box; repeat in reverse

Flutter kick w/kickboard, 1 lap on each of the 4 sides

Giant horizontal scissors kick w/kickboard, 30 face up, 30 face down

1 lap breaststroke kick

1 lap backward jog w/alternate punches to the front

45 jumping jacks, 45 leg swings each leg, 45 slaloms

30 jogs through tires

Double knee tucks in a box: 4 tucks pushing backward, then make 1/4 turn; 4 tucks and turn again, etc

Complete the box

For 4 sets: 8 side steps right, 3 hamstring curls, 8 side steps left, 3 hamstring curls

For 4 sets: alternate 8 small forward kicks w/4 giant forward kicks

COOL DOWN AND STRETCH

COMMENTS

Any reverse motion will burn slightly more calories than the same motion going forward. The reverse movements in this workout will improve balance and coordination while burning calories. Water-walk the two-step 1 lap forward, 1 backward.

WORKOUT 6

FORTY-SOMETHING
TIME: 40 minutes in THRZ

6

WARM-UP: Deep water

WORKOUT

Location: Deep water
Pace: Rhythmically
Effort: 3-4 RPE; 60-69% max HR
Activity:
Alternate each of the following with a 2-minute basic run:
40 side steps left, 40 right
40 vertical flutters
40 gallops
40 water polo goalie
40 forward abdominal crunches
40 prone horizontal scissors
40 abdominal crunches each side
40 cross-country ski
40 pistons
40 supine horizontal scissors

Repeat entire workout

COOL DOWN AND STRETCH

COMMENTS

Moving across the width of the deep end, up and back in a lane or in place, calculate about 40 steps of basic jog for 1 length.

WORKOUT 7

7

BUTT BURNER
TIME: 45-50 minutes

WARM-UP: A or B

WORKOUT

Location: Shallow water
Pace: Strong and firm
Effort: 3-4 RPE; 60-69% max HR
Activity:

Side lunges with shoulder scoops, 40 each way

40 easy jogs

Alternating side lunges, punching opposite arm, 40 each way

40 hard jogs

55 cross-country ski

50 wide jogs through tires

40 small kicks backward

40 small, tight jogs

50 pendulum kicks

40 jogs w/knees up high

40 slaloms

50 jogs w/jumping jack arms

Alternating legs, "kick yourself" 40 times

For 2 reps: 8 sideways jogs left, 8 right

50 giant kicks

40 easy jogs

Tuck and extend 40x each leg

50 double knee tucks wide to the side

Jog hard 40x

Alternate knee lift, crossing foot in front of other ankle

Repeat entire workout

COOL DOWN AND STRETCH

COMMENTS

This workout is focused on nonstop motion of the large muscles of the lower body.

WORKOUT 8

SPORTS CIRCUIT TRAINING
TIME: 38 minutes in THRZ

8

WARM-UP: A or B

WORKOUT

Location: Shallow water
Pace: Powerful
Effort: 3-4 RPE; 60-69% max HR
Activity:
At each station, repeat exercises 45 times, legs first, then arms
Station 1: alternate hamstring curl, figure-8 arms
Station 2: gallop sideways, butterfly-stroke arms
Station 3: power knee swing, breaststroke arms
Station 4: total-body twist, figure-8 arms
Station 5: rocking-horse, racquet swing
Station 6: cross-country ski, deep arm pulls
Station 7: jog through tires, upright row
Station 8: bob, backstroke arms
Station 9: jumping jacks, power punch

COOL DOWN slowly for 8 x 25 yards—your choice of movement
w/20-second rest intervals.

STRETCHES in water.

COMMENTS

Imagine yourself in a large athletic event, about to give your best
performance ever. Use an Aqua bar in each hand, webbed gloves, or
cupped hands against the direction of movement to increase upper-
body challenge.

9

HALF AND HALF
TIME: 38 minutes in THRZ

WARM-UP: A or B

WORKOUT

Location: Shallow water
Pace: Moderate
Effort: 3-4 RPE; 60-69% max HR
Activity:
2 laps each:
Freestyle, 45 bobs each lap
Backstroke, 40 jumping jacks each lap
Breaststroke, 50 pendulums each lap
Pull only, 75 fast jogs each lap
Your choice, 65 cross-country ski each lap
Kick only, 30 butterfly arms each lap
Freestyle, slalom 60 times each lap

Repeat all vertical motions back to back

COOL DOWN w/8 x 25 yards slow and steady your choice and 20-second rest intervals.

STRETCHES in water.

COMMENTS

This workout makes the transition from lengths to laps. A lap is usually 50 yards or meters.

WORKOUT 10

650-SWIM
TIME: 25-30 minutes

10

WARM-UP: B

WORKOUT

Location: Shallow or deep water
Pace: Constant and steady
Effort: 3-4 RPE; 60-69% max HR
Activity:
Bob 1 minute
50 yards slow swim, style of your choice
100 yards crawl
Rest 30 seconds
50 yards backstroke
50 yards crawl
100 yards breaststroke
50 yards crawl
100 yards breaststroke
50 yards kick only on your back
For 3 reps: 25 crawl, pull, kick, swim
50 yards backstroke
50 crawl

COOL DOWN with an easy kick medley, your choice.

STRETCHES in the water.

COMMENTS

Swimming on the back has the advantages of uninhibited breathing and increased workload for the legs.

Purple Zone

These short-duration workouts are composed of the same basic moves you have already mastered. You will be working at a steady pace, with less recovery time between intense moves. Purple workouts bring you into the moderate range of intensity.

WORKOUT 1

1

UPPER-BODY STRENGTH TRAINING
TIME: 30 minutes

WARM-UP: Both A and B

WORKOUT

Location: Shallow water
Pace: Fast and firm
Effort: 4-7 RPE; 70-79% max HR
Activity:

For 6 reps: feet astride, 4 punches down, 4 to side, 4 forward

For 6 reps: 4 big claps, 4 lateral raises, 4 biceps/triceps presses

Change feet to lunge, hands together. For 30 reps: punch forward, in front of hips; punch circling forward and down; reverse circle

For 45 reps: feet astride, lunge right, punching hands; lunge left

With abdominals tight, hands together, raise arms to the right corner, for 40 reps: push straight down between knees and pull straight up to the left corner, making a "V"

40 side-swing arms; 40 smaller swings double-time

Sit on flotation. Once balanced, raise hands to the surface. Breaststroke arms 1 length or 45x. Reverse. Canoe arms 1 length or 45x w/each arm as lead. Stay vertical and dog-paddle in a small circle 8 counts right, 8 left.

Bend knees to chest and place flotation under feet. Quickly extend legs pushing the flotation deeper for a quick lift. Repeat 30x or try the extension slow and controlled, balancing for 30 seconds.

COOL DOWN AND STRETCH

COMMENTS

Use your favorite piece of buoyant hand-held equipment: Aqua bars, Gyrojoggers, kickboards, or woggles. Elbows should push and pull widely. Keep knees astride or lunge to protect lower back.

WORKOUT 2

WATER EXERCISE PROGRESSIONS
TIME: 30 minutes

2

WARM-UP: A

WORKOUT

Location: Shallow water

Pace: Rebound, neutral, and suspended

Effort: 4-7 RPE; 70-79% max HR

Activity:

For each exercise, give 1 minute rebound, 1 minute neutral, 1 minute suspended:

Total-body twist

Bob

Slalom

Jog

Cross-country ski

Pendulum

Giant kick

Jumping jacks

Hamstring curls

Skip

COOL DOWN AND STRETCH

COMMENTS

A great workout if you are tired or stressed out. Have fun with this one!

WORKOUT 3

3

ALL-AMERICAN
TIME: 20 minutes in the THRZ

WARM-UP: A

WORKOUT

Location: Shallow water
Pace: Aggressive
Effort: 4-7 RPE; 70-79% max HR
Activity:

4 minutes water-walking

45 bobs

45 pendulums

30 double knee tucks

45 cross-country ski

30 slaloms

60 jogs through tires

30 hamstring curls alternating each side

30 giant kicks

Side step 2 laps or 8 right, 8 left for 4 reps

Tuck and extend 45x each leg

45 total-body twists

Rocking-horse 45x each leg

Flutter kick in all 4 directions using kickboard or the wall to support upper body, 1 lap each side or 1 minute each

60 jogs in place

45 jumping jacks, alternate arms crossing front and back

60 relaxed bobs

60 rear leg lifts alternating each side

COOL DOWN AND STRETCH

COMMENTS

Build stamina quickly with the 16 most popular shallow-water exercises used for aerobic conditioning. Your choice of arms makes for an invigorating top-to-bottom training.

WORKOUT 4

COMBINATIONS
TIME: 30 minutes

WARM-UP: A

WORKOUT

Location: Shallow water

Pace: Moderate and steady

Effort: 4-7 RPE; 70-79% max HR

Activity:

For 6 sets: 4 jumping jacks, 4 twists left, 4 diagonal kicks, 4 twists right.

For 4 sets, 2nd and 4th in the opposite order: 4 giant kicks, 4 double knee tucks, 4 alternate knee lifts, 4 alternate hamstring curls, 4 leg lifts in back.

For each set, decrease reps from 40-30-20-10-4 each: march, cross-country ski, bob (facing north, east, south, west), pendulum swings.

For 4 sets and leading with one leg: 8 leg lifts, 8 pendulums, 1/4 turn toward the free leg, 8 rocking-horses, 8 jogs. Repeat, leading with the other leg.

For 6 sets, leading with one leg: grapevine 8 counts to the side, 8 sideways slaloms, 8 front, 8 back. Tuck and extend outside leg 8x. Repeat, leading with the other leg.

COOL DOWN AND STRETCH

COMMENTS

Large-muscle-moving exercises are repeated in short but safe sequences. Done correctly, these are sure to keep you working hard the whole time.

WORKOUT 5

5

DEEP-WATER WORK
TIME: 30 minutes

WARM-UP: Deep water

WORKOUT

Location: Deep water

Pace: Deliberate

Effort: 4-7 RPE; 70-79% max HR

Activity:

Jog twice around a circle about 25 feet in diameter. Turn quickly to face your own eddy. Complete 1 more circle and turn. Jog a backward circle or 50 steps.

Repeat jog sequence after each of the following: cross-country ski 2 circles or 2 minutes; water polo goalie in place 1 minute; vertical flutter 1 minute; flick 1 minute.

While holding onto wall or flotation, 60 horizontal scissors prone, 60 supine; 60 abdominal crunches straight, 60 diagonal; 60 bicycles; 40 pendulums.

COOL DOWN AND STRETCH

COMMENTS

If you are new to deep water and feel yourself relaxing, visualize yourself actually running on a track. "Feel" the pavement under your front foot; push off with your back leg. The thrust of each leg will cause your shoulders to rise in the water. A flotation belt or Gyrojoggers are needed.

WORKOUT 6

FANTASTIC 50
TIME: 24 minutes in THRZ

6

WARM-UP: A or B

WORKOUT

Location: Shallow water
Pace: Deliberate and fast
Effort: 4-7 RPE; 70-79% max HR
Activity:
50 of each of the following for 2 sets:

Cross-country ski
Jog
Pendulum
Left leg swing
Right leg swing
Total-body twist
Knee tuck
Squat and lift
Left rocking-horse
Right rocking-horse

Lunge and punch alternating sides
Back leg lift
Bob
Hamstring curl
Tuck and extend left
Tuck and extend right
Jog hard
Slalom

COOL DOWN AND STRETCH

COMMENTS

Varied resistance to all the major muscle groups makes this a fast and efficient use of training time.

WORKOUT 7

7

SHALLOW-WATER DANCING
TIME: 18 minutes in THRZ

WARM-UP: A

WORKOUT

Location: Shallow water

Pace: Slow but powerful

Effort: 4-7 RPE; 70-79% max HR

Activity:

Pattern 1—For 4 sets, alternating lunge: 2 lunges and recovers w/deep pull arms; 4 marches w/power arms; 4 jogs forward w/figure-8 arms; 4 twists back w/big claps

Pattern 2—Repeat 4x to make a box w/right leg leading: 4 grapevines right; 4 jogs back w/biceps curl; 4 rocking-horses; 4 bobs; 1/4 turn right on 4th bob. Repeat, making a box w/left leg leading

Pattern 3—For 2 sets right, then 2 sets left: 1 jumping jack; 3 cross-country ski; 3 twists; 1 jumping jack; 2 side leaps; 2 hops back; 3 cross-country ski; 2 quick hops of 1/4 turn

Pattern 4—For 4 sets, alternating lead leg: 8 tuck and extends; 8 bobs; 8 slaloms; 8 twists

COOL DOWN AND STRETCH

COMMENTS

For a grand finale, repeat each pattern 1 time straight through.

WORKOUT 8

CIRCUIT TRAINING
TIME: 18 minutes in THRZ

8

WARM-UP: A

WORKOUT

Location: Shallow water
Pace: Intense
Effort: 4-7 RPE; 70-79% max HR
Activity:

Station 1: 8 sideways gallops right, 8 left for 3 reps; 40 giant scissors arms

Station 2: 40 straight leg swings right, 40 left; 30 canoe arms each side

Station 3: 40 double knee lifts; 20 biceps/triceps curls

Station 4: 50 pendulums; 40 straight arm circles each side

Station 5: 50 twists; 40 big claps

Station 6: 50 rocking-horses each leg; 40 deep pulls

Station 7: 50 tuck and extends; 40 power arms each arm

Station 8: 60 jogs; 30 bow-and-arrows each arm

Station 9: 50 jumping jacks; 50 lateral raises

Station 10: 50 cowboy jogs; 50 alternate punches up

Station 11: 50 alternating hamstring curls; 25 side swing arms

Station 12: 8 grapevine counts right, 8 left for 4 sets; biceps/triceps curls in varied positions

COOL DOWN AND STRETCH

COMMENTS

Combining the power of strength training with the endurance required for aerobic training creates a time-saving workout. Make sure small-muscle moves are intense enough to keep you in your THRZ.

WORKOUT 9

9

HALF AND HALF
TIME: 24 minutes in THRZ

WARM-UP: B

WORKOUT

Location: Shallow water
Pace: Faster than normal
Effort: 4-5 RPE; 70-79% max HR
Activity:

200-yard mixed WARM-UP: random pulls, kicks, swim any stroke

Between each of the vertical movements do 4 x 25, alternate easy and sprint

60 jumping jacks

60 double knee tucks

30 pendulums each side

60 slaloms

60 total-body twists

60 tuck and extends each side

60 jogs through tires

30 hamstring curls

COOL DOWN AND STRETCH

COMMENTS

Take rest intervals as needed. In smaller spaces, do 4 25-yard sprints between each exercise.

SWIM

TIME: 45-50 minutes

10

WARM-UP: B

WORKOUT

Location: Shallow water
Pace: 25-30 seconds per length
Effort: 3-4 RPE; 60-69% max HR
Activity:
For 2 reps: 50 yards easy; 50 yards kick; 50 yards pull
100 yards straight w/15-second rest
50 yards freestyle
50 yards backstroke
50 yards breaststroke
50 yards pull only
50 yards kick only
50 yards slow breaststroke
50 yards backstroke kick only
50 yards backstroke pull only
For 8 reps: push off w/prone glide, then dolphin kick across with
board

COOL DOWN AND STRETCH IN THE WATER

COMMENTS

This is an interval workout varying easy with hard tasks—the best
way to build endurance.

9

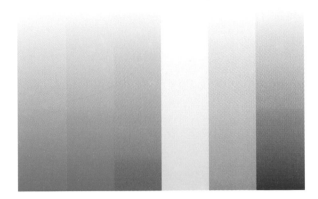

Yellow Zone

The Yellow zone is still very manageable for most people in terms of intensity. I think it depends on what you had for breakfast! You will be working at an intensity of about 4 to 7. Training heart rates approach 79 percent of your maximum. All Yellow workouts exceed the ACSM suggested minimum of 20 to 30 minutes within your THR. The increased length of time qualifies each as especially good fat-burning workouts. Maintaining this intensity for 30 to 45 minutes is an inspiring measure of your cardiovascular fitness.

1

WATER-WALKING

WATER-WALKING

TIME: 43 minutes in THRZ

WARM-UP: A or B

WORKOUT

Location: Shallow water
Pace: Sharp and crisp
Effort: 4-7 RPE; 70-85% max HR
Activity:

2 laps two-steps
2 laps twisting backward
4 laps skipping
2 laps bobbing backward
2 twists forward
1 lap jumping jacks
2 laps fast jogging
1 length jumping jacks, forward, backward and to sides
4 laps cross-country ski
2 laps double knee tucks going backward
2 laps fast jogging, pushing flotation out front

2 laps fast jogging, pulling flotation behind
2 laps skipping
1 side gallop w/right leg leading, 1 w/left
2 laps racquet swing
4 laps walking on water
2 laps cowboy jog
1 lap of 2 backward twists, 1 jumping jack
2 laps giant strides
2 laps rocking-horse
1 lap grapevine w/right leg leading, 1 w/left

COOL DOWN AND STRETCH

COMMENTS

You will need hand-held flotation to increase upper-body challenge.

LOWER-BODY SPORT SHAPE-UP

TIME: 40 minutes in THRZ

2

WARM-UP: A or B

WORKOUT

Location: Shallow water
Pace: Explosive
Effort: 4-7 RPE; 70-85% max HR
Activity:

50 run in place
50 leg swings each leg
50 jumping jacks inside only
60 cross-country ski
50 double knee tucks
60 diagonal kicks
60 pendulums
60 rear leg lifts
60 bobs north, south, east, west

60 fast jogs
60 easy jogs
60 total-body twists
For 10 reps: 4 sideways gallops right, 4 left
60 deep pulls
60 tuck and extends each leg
60 bobs

Repeat entire workout

COOL DOWN AND STRETCH

COMMENTS

Higher repetitions call for extra attention to proper form. Explosive moves that simulate sport actions build stamina in the lower body.

WORKOUT 3

3

TIME: 46 minutes

WARM-UP: Deep water

WORKOUT

Location: Deep water
Pace: Strong
Effort: 4-7 RPE; 70-85% max HR
Activity:
Do all of the following running in place:

2-3-minute easy run

2-minute cross-country ski

1-minute moderate run

1-minute fast run

2-minute cross-country ski

1-minute fast run

1-minute moderate run

1-minute vertical flutter

2-minute moderate run

For 4 reps: 30 fast run, 30 cross-country ski

1-minute moderate run

1-minute fast run

2-minute cross-country ski

1-minute fast run

1-minute moderate run

1-minute vertical flutter

1-minute moderate run

On the wall or w/equipment: 60 bicycles face up, 60 face down; 60 abdominal crunches and extends forward, 60 to each side

COOL DOWN AND STRETCH

COMMENTS

Add a tether to increase the intensity. Rest as needed for a few seconds, breathing deeply.

COMBINATIONS
TIME: 36 minutes in THRZ

4

WARM-UP: A or B

WORKOUT

Location: Shallow water
Pace: Moderately intense
Effort: 4-7 RPE; 70-80% max HR
Activity:

For 8 sets, alternating lead legs: 8 twists forward, 8 back; 8 lunges, punching alternate sides; 8 hamstring curls; 8 jogs through tires; 8 jumping jacks; 8 grapevines forward, diagonal right; 8 left side steps; 8 grapevines backward, diagonal right; 8 skips forward; 8 rocking-horses backward; 4 twists. Move through the set again and back again in reverse. Make a 1/4 turn and repeat sequence 3 more times.

For 4 sets each facing a different direction: 4 leg lifts in back, alternating legs; 4 hamstring curls; 8 fast jogs; 4 jogs through tires; 4 giant kicks; 8 side steps w/kick on 8th; 8 cross-country ski; 8 twists; 8 slaloms back and forth; 8 bobs

COOL DOWN AND STRETCH

COMMENTS

Feel the force of the water against your body as you turn, kick, and jump. Make your own tidal wave.

5

GYROJOGGER WORKOUT

TIME: 35 minutes in THRZ

WARM-UP: A or B

WORKOUT

Location: Shallow water

Pace: Energetic

Effort: 4-7 RPE; 70-85% max HR

Activity:

Place a Gyrojogger around each hand. While jogging, 8 power punches forward, 8 to alternating sides, 8 down. Repeat this jog and punch set each time you see "Gyro!"

60 twists w/Gyrojoggers by hips; 60 cross-country ski; Gyro!

60 pendulums; 60 double knee tucks w/jump rope arms; Gyro!

60 jumping jacks, straddle only; 60 hamstring curls; Gyro!

100 double knee tucks w/Gyrojoggers pushed down to knees and slightly forward while knees tuck, and land slightly toward the back; reverse pulling Gyrojoggers back, knees forward; 60 diagonal giant kicks; Gyro!

60 leg swings each leg; 60 jumping jacks; Gyro!

60 tuck and extends each leg; 60 power jogs; Gyro!

45 skips in place

Double knee tucks w/knees wide to the side, working Gyrojoggers down low by the hips

Repeat entire workout

COOL DOWN AND STRETCH

COMMENTS

You can adjust the intensity by how far under the water you keep your hands.

WORKOUT 6

60-SECOND STORM

TIME: 48 minutes in THRZ

WARM-UP: A or B

WORKOUT

Location: Shallow water

Pace: Varied intensity

Effort: 4-7 RPE; 70-85% max HR

Activity:

Each time you see the word "storm," jog fast and tight in place as if you were a child having a tantrum. Use your arms powerfully, splashing with the elbows to make a blizzard. Your intense storm should last around 60 seconds. Then do 60 squat and lifts.

60 rocking-horses left, 60 right; Storm!

60 moderate jogs; 60 tuck and extends left, 60 right; Storm!

60 pendulums; 60 bobs w/knees wide; Storm!

60 cross-country ski; 60 double knee tucks; Storm!

60 giant kicks forward; 60 kicks diagonal; Storm!

60 slaloms; 60 jumping jacks; Storm!

60 twists; 60 leg swings left, 60 right; Storm!

Repeat entire workout

COOL DOWN AND STRETCH

COMMENTS

Guaranteed to rid you of frustration.

7

DEEP-WATER PARTNERS

DEEP-WATER PARTNERS

TIME: 46 minutes

WARM-UP: Deep water

WORKOUT

Location: Shallow water
Pace: Sharp and crisp
Effort: 4-7 RPE; 70-80% max HR
Activity:

Use a partner and a flotation belt.

1-minute backward run side-by-side

30 side steps each direction

2-minute moderate run

1-minute back-to-back flutter kick

60 jumping jacks

20 pendulums

1-minute vertical flutter

2-minute prone hand-to-hand flutter

Swing your partner 2x each arm

2-minute moderate run

2-minute cross-country ski

1-minute back-to-back flutter kick

60 angels in the snow

1-minute flicking

2-minute back-to-back flutters

2-minute moderate run

2-minute cross-country ski

2-minute vertical flutter

Swing your partner 2x each way

Swim 1 length, partner holding your ankles, while you do arm strokes, partner kicks, then trade places 1 length

Repeat sequence

End with 70 tucks, 70 diagonal tucks, 70 pendulums

COOL DOWN AND STRETCH

COMMENTS

Working with a partner adds extra resistance. Keep a safe distance when jogging or kicking, but close enough to cause some turbulence for each other.

CIRCUIT

TIME: 40 minutes in THRZ

WARM-UP: A or B

WORKOUT

Location: Shallow water

Pace: Animated

Effort: 4-7 RPE; 70-85% max HR

Activity:

Station 1:	1-minute bobbing in place; 1-minute punches forward w/alternating arms
Station 2:	60 jogs through tires; biceps/triceps curls
Station 3:	8 sideways gallops right, 8 left; repeat 4x; 60 lateral arm raises crossing in front
Station 4:	60 cross-country ski; 30 side arm circles left, 30 right
Station 5:	50 straight leg swings left, 50 right; 60 lateral arm raises crossing in back
Station 6:	60 leg lifts rearward w/alternating legs; 60 big claps
Station 7:	60 total-body twists, big and powerful; 50 deep arm pulls
Station 8:	40 hamstring curls each alternating side; 60 canoe arms

Repeat all 8 stations with a 45-second jog in between

COOL DOWN AND STRETCH

COMMENTS

Have fun exaggerating the moves. Use with Gyrojoggers, webbed gloves, or Aqua bars.

9

HALF AND HALF

TIME: 41 minutes in THRZ

WARM-UP: A or B

WORKOUT

Location: Shallow water
Pace: Vigorous
Effort: 4-7 RPE; 70-85% max HR
Activity:

50 yards freestyle

60 cross-country ski

2 x 50 back crawl

60 rocking-horses

3 x 75 your choice—pull, kick, swim—anything but crawl

60 tuck and extends

3 x 75 breaststroke pull, kick, swim

60 jumping jacks, straddle only

4 x 50 back-breast

100 bobs

6 x 50 crawl

60 double knee tucks

3 x 75 back pull, kick, swim

100 slaloms

100 sprints

60 giant kicks

5 minutes your choice (easy)

COOL DOWN AND STRETCH

COMMENTS

Reduce rest periods by using the vertical time to breathe deeply. Keep activities continuous throughout workout.

1575-YARD SWIM

TIME: 36 minutes in THRZ

10

WARM-UP: B

WORKOUT

Location: Shallow or deep water

Pace: Constant and steady

Effort: 4-7 RPE; 70-85% max HR

Activity:

Use webbed gloves:

2 laps easy pace—your choice

3 x 50 easy pace—pull, kick, swim each for crawl, breaststroke, backstroke; 50-yard sprint; 100-yard crawl

4 x 100 breaststroke, rest interval (R.I.) 20 seconds

3 x 100 crawl, R.I. 20 seconds

1 x 100 25 your choice, 25 backstroke, 25 breaststroke, 25 crawl, R.I. 10 seconds; repeat the 100, kick only

Remove gloves:

50-yard scull w/kick; 100-yard sprint

3 x 50 backstroke, 50 left arm only, 50 right, 50 both

4 x 25 flutter kick on front, sides, back

5-minute treading in deep water

4-minute easy swim—your choice

70 tucks, 70 diagonal tucks, 70 pendulums

COOL DOWN AND STRETCH IN WATER

COMMENTS

Hand paddles or webbed gloves create resistance or drag in the water. They can also increase the perception of hand movements.

10

Orange Zone

Orange zone workouts are designed to push your body hard. Mentally you should aim for at least 90 percent of what you arc capable of doing. Engage the heart and lungs at a high intensity for a short period of timc. It feels good!

WORKOUT 1

1

WATER-WALKING WORKOUT
TIME: 45 minutes

WARM-UP: A

WORKOUT

Location: Shallow water
Pace: Powerful
Effort: 6-8 RPE; 80-95% max HR
Activity:
1 lap march w/triceps press
2 laps jogging backward w/power punches
1 lap jumping jacks forward
1 lap two-step w/canoe arms
1 lap skipping w/power arms
1 lap hard run
1 lap easy run
2 laps hard run
1 lap easy run
3 laps hard run

COOL DOWN AND STRETCH

COMMENTS

Midway into this training session, you will begin an intense pyramid. Once you reach the max, you then descend in increments to the minimum.

WORKOUT 2

SPORT SAMPLER
TIME: 35 minutes

WARM-UP: 2 laps water-walking forward, backward, sideways. Jog full speed, arms dragging behind. Jog backward, arms dragging in front. Calf stretch, quad stretch.

WORKOUT

Location: Shallow water

Pace: Powerful

Effort: 5-8 RPE; 70-95% max HR

Activity: Spend about 5 minutes "playing" each of the following sports:

Football: jog through tires 8 forward, 8 sideways, 8 backward, 8 in a circle; repeat set 5x; face partner, yell and charge; bump alternate shoulders 30 seconds; 50-yard quarterback run

Basketball: short sprints back and forth, decreasing yardage, then increasing; jumpshots w/partner's arms a basket; 20 hops on 1 foot, 20 on the other, 20 on both, 1 lap bobbing backward, 1 lap twisting backward

Karate: high sideways kick; 60 each leg—knee up, extend, pull down; 1-minute hamstring curls w/elbow pullback; 1-minute giant kicks; 1-minute diagonal kicks; 1 lap racquet kick

Tennis: 5 forehands, 5 backhands, alternating, weak arm first; repeat 5 sets

1-minute slalom; 2-minute 8 gallops right, 8 left; big jumps; high-5 a partner; lateral hop countdown from 10

Baseball: 10 swings full range of motion, left then right; "Got-cha-last." Fast run on lane line to tag a partner who turns around and tries to tag you back; change places; catch the fly ball; run bases; 2 circles around pool's perimeter; grapevines 8 right, 8 left for 6 sets

Skiing: 2-minute cross-country ski; 1-minute slalom; lunge forward, recover 60x; 20 360-degree turns

COOL DOWN AND STRETCH

COMMENTS

Use real sports equipment if you have old pieces no longer in use. Use your imagination! Work with a friend.

3

WATER BOXING
TIME: 28 minutes in THRZ

WARM-UP: A or B

WORKOUT

Location: Shallow water

Pace: Powerful

Effort: 5-8 RPE; 70-95% max HR

Activity:

Do 1 each of the following classic punching sets. Then, alternate punching sets with 3-minute rounds of typical boxers' aerobic conditioning, such as jogging in place, hopping, jumping rope, squatting and lifting, swinging legs.

Sets:

Left jab, right jab

Right jab, left hook

3 right jabs

Left jab, right upper cut

Left jab, right jab, left hook

Left upper cut, right jab

Left jab, right upper cut, left hook

Right hook, left upper cut

Left jab, right jab, left upper cut

Left jab, right hook

COOL DOWN AND STRETCH

WORKOUT 4

COMBINATIONS
TIME: 30 minutes in THRZ

WARM-UP: A

WORKOUT

Location: Shallow water

Pace: Powerful

Effort: 5-8 RPE; 70-95% max HR

Activity:

For 6 sets: 4 deep arm pulls bobbing forward; jog back 8; 8 straddle-only jumping jacks; 8 giant kicks; 8 pendulums

For 5 sets: 4 twists up, 4 back; 8 lunges, punching alternate sides; 8 hamstring curls; 4 rocking-horses left, 4 right

8 left leg forward tuck and extends; bob back 8; 8 right leg forward tuck and extends; bob back 8; straddle-only cross-country ski 8 w/left leg lead, 8 w/right

For 5 sets: 10 power jogs; 10 diagonal giant kicks; 10 small forward kicks; 10 straddle-only jumping jacks

For 5 sets: 8 squat and lifts alternate legs; 4 gallops right, 4 left; 4 double knee tucks; 4 straddle-only cross-country ski

COOL DOWN AND STRETCH

COMMENTS

These combinations take about 10 minutes each. Repeat 3 times through.

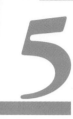

DEEP-WATER INTERVAL WORKOUT
TIME: 36 minutes in THRZ

WARM-UP: Deep water

WORKOUT

Location: Deep water
Pace: Powerful
Effort: 5-8 RPE; 70-85% max HR
Activity:

5-minute basic run at 70%
1-minute water polo goalie
4-minute basic run at 80%
1-minute vertical flutter
3-minute basic run at 85%
1-minute piston power, shaking shoulders hard
2-minute basic run at 80%
1-minute bouncy gallop

1-minute basic run at 80%
All sprints back-to-back
1-minute water polo goalie
1-minute vertical flutter
1-minute piston
1-minute gallop
2-minute basic run at 70%
1-minute gallop
5-minute basic run at 75%

COOL DOWN AND STRETCH

COMMENTS

Be sure to breathe deeply during runs. Wear a flotation device.

WORKOUT 6

DEEP-AND-SHALLOW WORKOUT

TIME: 32 minutes

WARM-UP: A

WORKOUT

Location: Shallow and deep water

Pace: Powerful

Effort: 5-8 RPE; 70-95% max HR

Activity:

Choose a pool lane that goes from shallow to deep. Begin with the first shallow-water activity. As you reach deep water change to the first deep-water activity to the end and back until your feet touch. Alternate between the following deep and shallow moves—about 1 minute each.

Shallow: bob; slalom; leg swing; twist; squat and lift; rocking-horse; tuck and extend; deep pull

Deep: jog; cross-country ski; vertical flutter; water polo goalie; piston; jumping jacks; flicking; crawl

Repeat entire workout

COOL DOWN AND STRETCH

COMMENTS

Move in place to complete an activity if needed. A combination of deep and shallow water workouts improves flexibility and strength.

WORKOUT 7

7

GET THOSE GLUTEALS
TIME: 35 minutes

WARM-UP: A or B

WORKOUT

Location: Deep water
Pace: Tight and strong
Effort: 5-8 RPE; 70-85% max HR
Activity:
60 giant kicks forward to corners, emphasizing pull down
60 pendulums
60 jogs through tires
30 jogs w/knees high
30 jogs w/heels up in back
6 reps of: 4 jogs w/knees high; 4 w/heels up
Double knee tucks
For 3 sets: 60 bobs; 60 skips; 30 leg swings each side; 60 rocking-horses each side; 30 back leg lifts each side
80 tucks; 80 diagonal tucks; 80 pendulums

COOL DOWN AND STRETCH

COMMENTS

Use firm, controlled movements to get the maximum strength-building benefits from this total-body workout. If you have back trouble, substitute different exercises for positions that place the heels behind the gluteals.

WORKOUT 8

SPORTS CIRCUITS
TIME: 32 minutes in THRZ

WARM-UP: A or B

WORKOUT

Location: Shallow water
Pace: Vigorous
Effort: 5-8 RPE; 70-85% max HR
Activity:

Station 1: fast jog 1 lap forward, 1 backward; 60 alternating arms racquet swing

Station 2: 60 straddle-only jumping jacks; 60 upright rows

Station 3: single leg swings, 60 each leg; 60 deep arm pulls

Station 4: 60 double knee tucks; 40 triceps extensions

Station 5: 60 pendulums; 60 lateral arm raises crossing in back

Station 6: 60 jogging through tires; 120 alternate punches down at sides

Station 7: 60 alternate straight leg lifts to the back; 60 lateral arm raises crossing in back

Station 8: 60 explosive slaloms; 60 power punches

COOL DOWN AND STRETCH

COMMENTS

You may use Aqua blocks or other hand-held resistance equipment.

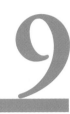

9

HALF AND HALF
TIME: 30 minutes

WARM-UP: 1-minute bob w/butterfly arms pulling you forward, then backward. 3-minute easy swim.

WORKOUT

Location: Deep water
Pace: Powerful
Effort: 5-8 RPE; 70-95% max HR
Activity:
3 x 150 alternate pull, kick, swim
2-minute deep-water run
2 x 200 alternate 2 backstroke; 2 breaststroke
2-minute water polo goalie
3 x 125 alternate slow, medium, fast crawls
2-minute gallop
1 x 200 easy swim, breathing on weak side
2-minute treading water, varying arms
80 tucks
80 diagonal tucks
80 pendulums

COOL DOWN AND STRETCH

COMMENTS

Equally balances upper- and lower-body strengthening.

SWIM

TIME: 35-40 minutes

WARM-UP: 1-minute bob; 1 x 25 each scull, backstroke, breaststroke, dolphin kick

WORKOUT

Location: Shallow or deep water
Pace: Powerful
Effort: 5-8 RPE; 70-95% max HR
Activity:
2 x 200 crawl, alternating breathing sides; R.I. 20 seconds
6 x 50, 2 pulls, 2 kicks, 2 swim
1 x 600 mixer (choose variation for each 50)
8 x 25 sprint
1 x 150 easy swim—your choice
2-minute treading water

COOL DOWN AND STRETCH

COMMENTS

With the mixer, you can do any stroke or combination of strokes except the crawl.

11

Red Zone

This is it! This is where you give it all you've got! These workouts are geared to get your heart rate up to 85-95 percent and to keep you in your training zone for up to 50 minutes. The challenge of the Red zone is to maintain the pace without reducing quality in the way you execute the moves. Participating in workouts of high intensity and long duration such as these requires that you are in great shape already and that you plan for appropriate rest days. Challenge yourself occasionally to continue to make fitness gains.

WORKOUT 1

1

WATER-WALKING
TIME: 60 minutes in THRZ

WARM-UP: A

WORKOUT

Location: Shallow water
Pace: Powerful
Effort: 8-9 RPE; 80-95% max HR
Activity:

1-minute pedal
1 lap two-step
1 lap forward lunge and recover
1 lap side step left, 1 right
2 laps easy jog
2 laps racquet swing
3 laps moderate jog
1 lap cross-country ski
2 laps walk on water
1 lap total-body twist backward
2 laps fast jog with crawl-stroke arms
1 lap jog through tires with funky arms forward, 1 backward
3 laps moderate jog

1 lap bobbing backward
1 lap knee swing left, 1 right
1 lap side gallops left, 1 right
1 lap hamstring curls moving forward w/deep pull arms
2 laps walking on water
1 lap forward jumping jacks
3 laps skipping
1 lap bobbing forward w/deep pulls
2 laps giant kicks forward moving backward w/ canoe arms
2 laps moderate jog
2 laps power walk

Repeat entire workout

COOL DOWN AND STRETCH

COMMENTS

The workout provides a few recovery laps, but the bulk of the water-walking should be done full speed ahead.

WORKOUT 2

WATER BOXING
TIME: 48 minutes in THRZ

2

WARM-UP: A or B

WORKOUT

Location: Shallow water

Pace: Fast and precise

Effort: 8-9 RPE; 80-95% max HR

Activity:

Repeat these classic punches 6 times: left jab, right jab, left hook, right hook, left upper cut, right upper cut.

For 7 sets, alternate the following 3-minute punching rounds with 3 minutes of cardiovascular training activities. Round 1: left jab, right jab. Round 2: right jab, left hook. Round 3: 3 right jabs. Round 4: left jab, right jab, left hook. Round 5: left jab, right upper cut. Round 6: right jab, left hook, left jab, right hook. Round 7: left jab, left hook, right jab, left hook. Round 8: left upper hook, right jab. Round 9: left hook, right hook, left hook, right hook, left upper cut, right jab. Round 10: left jab, right upper cut, left hook, left jab, right jab, left hook, right hook

COOL DOWN AND STRETCH

COMMENTS

Good cardiovascular activities to use are bob; jog through tires—left, right, front, back; jump rope—fast and small, slow and wide; power jog; gallop sideways; giant kicks. Use Gyrojoggers, Aqua bars, Bemas, or webbed gloves.

WORKOUT 3

3

DEEP-WATER TONING
TIME: 52 minutes in THRZ

WARM-UP: Deep water

WORKOUT

Location: Deep water

Pace: Full speed, forceful

Effort: 8-10 RPE; 80-95% max HR

Activity: Each set is done 7x, using these different arm movements for each rep: power pump, breaststroke, crawl stroke, biceps curl, lateral triceps press, rear triceps press, double arm pulls

Set 1: basic jog in a circle of about 18 x 25 feet across, changing direction at the end of each circle

Set 2: flutter kick face down from edge to center of circle; recover quickly to vertical w/double knee tuck; extend legs forward as if sitting in a chaise; flutter backward to circle edge

Set 3: cross-country ski back and forth from edge to center

Set 4: move in a circle in the sitting position, thighs parallel to the floor, using lower leg to propel you backward and forward

Repeat entire workout

STRETCH IN DEEP WATER

COMMENTS

Abdominals work nonstop as stabilizers during this workout. Speed is not as important as how much muscle and water you move.

COMBINATIONS
TIME: 52 minutes in THRZ

4

WARM-UP: A or B

WORKOUT

Location: Shallow water

Pace: Vigorous

Effort: 8-10 RPE; 80-95% max HR

Activity: Do this 1-minute kick combination between each set, alternating legs: knee up center and down; knee up across your body and down; straight leg swing forward, backward, forward, down

Set 1 for 8 reps: 8 hard jogs; 8 straddle-only jumping jacks; 8 double hamstring curls; 8 skip in place

Set 2 for 8 reps, alternating legs: 1 jumping jack; 3 cross-country ski; 3 twists; 1 jumping jack; 2 leaps left; 2 backward hops; 3 cross-country ski; 2 hops w/1/4 turn

Set 3 for 8 reps, alternating lead legs: 8 forward right diagonal grapevines; 8 side steps left; 8 backward right diagonal grapevines; 8 skips forward; 8 double knee tucks back; 4 twists

Set 4 for 8 reps each leg: 8 tuck and extends right; 8 side steps right; 8 straddle-only cross-country ski; 8 jogs

Set 5 for 8 reps: 8 forward jumping jacks; 2 double knee tucks each direction; 8 slaloms w/funky arms; 8 bobs w/deep pulls backward

Set 6 for 8 reps making a box facing in, then out: 4 gallops w/1/4 turn; 4 slaloms sideways, 4 front and back; 4 giant kicks; 8 small kicks

Set 7 for 4 reps: 8 jogs right, 8 left; 8 giant kicks backward diagonal; 8 twists; 8 hamstring curls alternating legs; 8 bobs forward

COOL DOWN AND STRETCH

COMMENTS

Do entire workout twice, cutting down the pattern numbers by half the second time.

5

DEEP-WATER CIRCUITS
TIME: 48 minutes in THRZ

WARM-UP: Deep water

WORKOUT

Location: Deep water

Effort: 7-9 RPE; 80-95% max HR

Activity:

Jog hard 90 seconds between stations if working with a group, or in place if alone

Do 3 minutes (or 200 reps) at each station

Station 1: cross-country ski with deep pulls

Station 2: pistons w/power arms

Station 3: alternate abdominal tucks w/diagonal extensions, arms moving opposite legs

Station 4: deep-water jumping jacks w/lateral raises in opposition

Station 5: water polo goalie

Station 6: abdominal tucks w/big clap arms

Station 7: vertical flutter

Station 8: vertical double knee tucks w/lateral arm raises in opposition

Station 9: gallop

Repeat entire workout

COOL DOWN AND STRETCH

COMMENTS

Try using Gyrojoggers or webbed gloves.

WORKOUT 6

TOTAL-BODY EXERCISE
TIME: 44 minutes in THRZ

6

WARM-UP: A or B

WORKOUT

Location: Shallow water

Pace: Vigorous

Activity:

70 reps of each: deep pulls; squat and lifts alternating left and right; twists; rocking-horses alternating left and right; straddle-only jumping jacks w/arms crossing in back; slaloms; hard jogs; straddle-only cross-country ski left; straddle-only cross-country ski right; tuck and extends left; tuck and extends right; straddle-only jumping jacks, arms crossing in front; bobs; small forward kicks; sideways gallops left; sideways gallops right; alternating hamstring curls; straddle-only jumping jacks; jogs through tires; hard jogs; pendulums; alternating leg swings; moderate jogs. Finish w/100 tucks, 100 diagonal tucks, 100 pendulums.

COOL DOWN AND STRETCH

COMMENTS

A great workout if you're about to enter competition in any sport, and want to avoid overuse injuries.

WORKOUT 7

7

BUTT BURNER
TIME: 54 minutes

WARM-UP: Deep water

WORKOUT

Location: Deep water
Pace: Varied
Effort: 7-9 RPE; 80-95% max HR
Activity:
2-minute basic jog
1-minute firm flutter kick each direction
1-minute treading water
80 giant kicks forward
1-minute jog
2-minute vertical flutter
60 cross-country ski
1-minute hard flutter kick each direction
1-minute treading water, hands up
60 horizontal giant scissors, supine
1-minute jog
60 horizontal giant scissors, nearly prone
60 cross-country ski

Repeat entire sequence 3x

Finish w/100 tucks, 100 diagonal tucks, 100 pendulums

COOL DOWN AND STRETCH

COMMENTS

For second rep, try to get your body high out of the water. For third, stay low and increase range of motion slightly without losing intensity.

WORKOUT 8

DECATHLON
TIME: 58 minutes in THRZ

8

WARM-UP: A or B

WORKOUT

Location: Shallow and deep water
Pace: Varied
Effort: 7-9 RPE; 90-100% max HR
Activity:

400-meter flat race

For 2 reps: 16 laps running in shallow lanes; 2 laps running broad jumps

While circling in place, 30 shot puts left, 30 right

High jump

100-meter flat race — 2 laps or 2 minutes tethered

While circling in shallow water, 20 discus left, 20 right

110 hurdles over 2 laps

2 laps pole vaulting

2-minute javelin throw, running and throwing to alternate sides

1500-meter race w/flotation belt for 60 laps or 30 minutes in shallow lanes

COOL DOWN AND STRETCH

COMMENTS

Be sure to extend your follow-through to full range of motion with shot put, discus, and javelin throw. Simulate throws with the weight of the water. Work both arms to achieve body symmetry. Timing for broad jump, hurdle, etc.—1 . . . 2. . .3 . . . go!

WORKOUT 9

9

SWIM-SWIM
TIME: 46 minutes

WARM-UP: Deep water

WORKOUT

Location: Deep water
Pace: Varied
Effort: 7-9 RPE; 80-95% max HR
Activity:

4 x 50 slow swim, your choice, R.I. 15 seconds at 100

2 x 100 each: freestroke, backstroke, breaststroke

4 x 50 each: R.I. 15 seconds at 50: backstroke, breaststroke, kick only, dolphin, backstroke, breaststroke, freestroke

3 x 25 each: crawl—pull, kick, and swim (P,K,S); breaststroke P,K,S; backstroke P,K,S; your choice P,K,S

COOL DOWN w/100 easy kick medley. 100 easy swim.
STRETCHES in water

COMMENTS

Try to polish your stroke for improved speed. Record your times for comparison.

THE MIXER
TIME: 50-60 minutes

WARM-UP: A or B

WORKOUT

Pace: Full-speed

Effort: 8-10 RPE; 90-100% max HR

Activity:

1-minute bob w/butterfly arms

3 x 200 crawl

R.I 45 seconds

2 x 50 each: crawl, breaststroke, backstroke, your choice

8 x 100 drill: See how many strokes you take from one end to the other; reduce the number of strokes by 1 on the way back

400 kicks on back w/fins

200 swim

200 easy kick medley

COOL DOWN AND STRETCH

COMMENTS

Your attention here should be half on quality strokes and half on quantity.

PART III

TRAINING BY THE WORKOUT ZONES

Continued good health and satisfaction with your fitness aquatics program requires that you always have options to match your current abilities and ambitions. You've learned how to work the water and you've sampled the many combinations and styles of exercises that lead to improved health. Part III extends these concepts, encouraging you to construct the workout program that fulfills your needs, as you move through different stages of your life.

The color-coded workout zones encourage you to mix zones many ways. Every athlete or exerciser can incorporate all the zones into a training schedule. For example, graduated Green and Blue zone workouts interspersed with Purple zone workouts work well for recreational sport enthusiasts and post-competition athletes. Chapter 12 points out the importance of rest and nutrition to your feelings of well-being. Chapter 13 offers sample programs that have been successful for others. Chapter 14 discusses cross-training options and ways to spice up your favorite workouts. Chapter 15 closes with different approaches to charting and evaluating your progress. A blank form is provided for you to record your accomplishments.

12

Setting Up Your Program

Fitness is a package deal. If your focus has always been weight training and you do nothing to develop aerobic capacity, you do not have overall fitness. Likewise, having a strong heart and lungs is great, but you need power and flexibility as well. Elite athletes have a coach or trainer who creates a training plan; your training depends on how well *you* plan, set goals, and then stick to your plan. Focus on where you want to be fitness-wise and decide on a step-by-step method to achieve your goal. Include in your plans a balance of all the physical fitness components discussed in chapter 1. As you target your weak spots for improvement, don't forget to maintain your strengths.

Progression

Progression is how fast you reach your desired level of fitness. Taking on too much too soon is the number-one reason people fail to stick with a fitness program. Rushing can lead to soreness, injury, and excessive fatigue. A much better choice is to start slow and easy. Listen to your body. Are you breathing enough to supply the oxygen needed for the

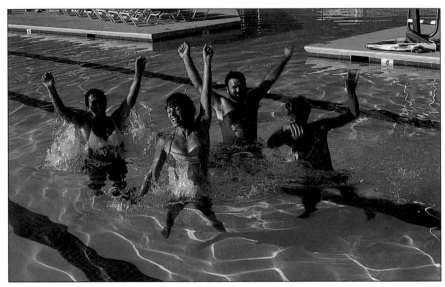

Fitness aquatics is a social activity.

working muscles? Focus on posture, form, and the finer points of each exercise. Make sure the muscle you want to contract is the one doing the work. Are you having fun yet?

The initial phase of an aquatic fitness program, which may last from one week to two months, involves getting accustomed to the activity, the shoes, the waves, and the new equipment. Work out any kinks, and use workouts in the Green and Blue zones to build a foundation of fitness.

When you feel working within these zones is not demanding enough, you are ready to give your body a challenge. Looking at the fitness variables of frequency, intensity, and time (F.I.T.), choose only one F.I.T. variable and increase it by about 10 percent. From the Purple or Yellow zone, find a workout that increases your time in the training zone. Work at that level until it is very comfortable. Next, you might choose the same workout but push harder to improve strength and keep your heart rate a bit higher. Increasing the demands on your body with a goal in mind is known as the "improvement phase" of training. It usually lasts 2 to 10 months, depending on your personal goals.

The final phase of progression is called maintenance. Keep things interesting and use a variety of workouts similar to those that helped get you into good shape. You'll be adding workouts from the Orange and Red zones. Continue to work in all the different color zones; each has unique benefits and foci. At least once a week, challenge yourself and include something more intense than usual.

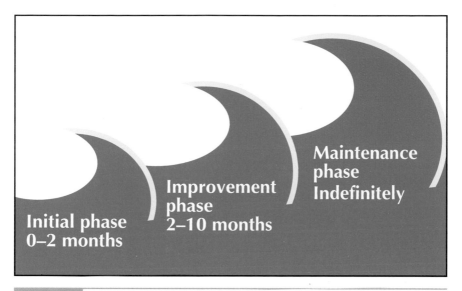

Figure 12.1 Staircase of progression

Reversibility of Training

Fitness declines quickly if activity stops. For inactive people, muscle mass, metabolism, strength, and aerobic conditioning decline at a rate of about 18 percent a year after the age of 30. You can maintain what you have fought for with three workouts per week. The secret is to develop fitness habits that are efficient and so enjoyable that you can continue for a lifetime.

Planning a 12-Month Program

"Periodization" is a term used to describe the grouping of months into a year-long training cycle. The four classic seasons used by competition-class athletes, equally applicable and beneficial to noncompetitors, are early season, refinement season, competition time, and active recovery. Each season takes a different approach to the training. This seasonal approach is a way to plan your workouts for definite progress, variety, and reduced chance of overuse injury.

- **Early**—prepare yourself for what is to come. Keep everything low-key, and build slowly. For 6 to 12 weeks, focus on the basic skills you'll be using and on flexibility.
- **Refinement**—preseason work focuses on perfecting technique. Build slowly, using the Yellow and Orange zones, and moderate

repetitions with moderate resistance. Continue the gradual increase in power and strength for about 18 weeks. This is a good time to add equipment.

- **Competition**—this peak season means continuous high-intensity workouts from the Orange and Red zones, with quality recovery days in Yellow, Purple, Blue, and Green zones. Incorporate specialized workouts (like the Orange zone's Sports Circuits #8) to develop speed and agility. Competition time is tough, usually lasting 8 to 14 weeks.
- **Active Recovery**—maintain your fitness with less intense workouts. Do some mental exploring and plan new things you would like to try for the upcoming year. Recovery season lasts about four weeks.

Overload

Improvement comes when the body is regularly stimulated beyond its normal workload. Physically, overloading challenges the body; growth and adaptations ensure that the body can better meet a similar demand next time. If you want growth, overload should be applied in each of the F.I.T. variables discussed in chapter 1. For swimmers, this method is called over-distance training. If you're in training for a 400m freestyle, practice a lot of 800m-to-1500m swims. Runners might take a look at the Decathlon workout in Red zone #8. The increased weight and drag of the water cause overload to the muscles, the improvement makes a race on land seem more manageable. Often overload is just giving one more repetition when you think you can do no more.

Rest

I remember a professor telling of a track team practice when all members were asked to run their all-time best. The coach wanted to see 120 percent effort from each team member. Times were recorded; everyone ran hard and gave a stellar performance. At the next practice, the coach asked them to run a little easier. Everyone ran at about 90 percent effort, and times were compared. They had all bettered their time from the previous day! What was the difference? Tension, pressure, and stress interfere with work between muscle pairs. While one is contracting, the other must relax. Tension reduces speed, blood flow, and overall performance (not to mention increasing pain and discomfort). Rest is necessary before, during, and after exercise. Any body part must have recovery time to rebuild and get prepared for the next challenging workout. The basic principle is to let the primary muscle group rest 48 hours before working it hard again. Don't be inactive, but change the focus elsewhere on the body. This alternating hard vs. easy concept lends variety and gives your body the rest it deserves. Target your upper body during one workout, followed by lower-body or aerobic emphasis during the next. If you swim or exercise faster, harder, or longer than usual one day, schedule an easy day from a Blue, Green, or Purple zone for your next day or two.

The first twinge of pain should never be ignored—it is your body's request for rest. As a general rule, I give myself three days with modified activity when I have a new pain. If the pain subsides, I carry on. If after three days the condition is unchanged or worse, or reoccurs from time to time, off to the doctor I go. The earlier you catch a problem, the less severe it will be. This tenet is especially true for swimmers, who risk overuse injury in the shoulder area. If you sense the need for a rest in any body part, but still want exercise, choose a workout that will maintain your cardiovascular level without stressing that one muscle group or joint: boxing, Gyrojogger or deep-water workouts won't aggravate pain in the knee or ankle; water-walking is a great alternative if you are nursing an upper-body injury.

If injuries are a recurring problem, evaluate your technique, posture, equipment, and rest habits. A different hand or foot position can engage entirely different muscles. Possibly your workouts are too long or intense. Our bodies are amazingly resilient. With appropriate variations your workouts can usually continue.

Relaxation is a word which should be in everyone's vocabulary. Relaxing just after the workout allows oxygen-laden blood to permeate the muscles. Relaxation offers a wonderful contrasting sensation after working vigorously.

Eating Smart!

A smart eating plan can also help achieve fitness. Practice an improved eating plan for at least three days. Notice whether it affects your performance, attitude, and wellness. Some people will respond more quickly than others to dietary changes but good nutrition will eventually result in your looking and feeling vibrant.

Reducing calories with restrictive diets slows the metabolic rate, while frequent workouts raise the metabolism. A person intent on lowering body fat is more likely to see results quickly with twice-a-day workouts of short duration combined with a smart eating plan. A plan that encompasses *both* exercise and moderate changes in calories consumed will be the most successful at maintaining lean body tissue and getting rid of the fat.

The body loses fluids even while in the water. People still sweat during aerobic workouts in the water. Hydrostatic pressure exerts force from all direction on each cell, squeezing out excess liquid. (That is why one hour in the pool will usually eliminate any swelling.) The best choice for replacing liquid is water, which is most quickly absorbed. Second choice is fruit juices. Alcohol and caffeine are nowhere on the list, because they cause further dehydration. If you are in a hot room or in warmer water, you should have small sips of cool liquid every 10 to 15 minutes throughout the workout. In one study of the effects of water temperature on the body's absorption rate, ice-water was absorbed twice as fast as warm water. Cold liquids also help reduce the core temperature of the body, and prevent overheating.

13

Sample Aquatic Programs

Training programs are as varied as their participants. And there's bound to be a good fit for you. Continue to mix and match until you find a comfortable routine that propels you toward your goals. Here are some suggested schedules for three different fitness levels: beginning, moderate, and intense. Within each schedule you'll find the training principles discussed in earlier chapters. As you tailor your training program, be sure to consider progression, overload, F.I.T., and rest.

Beginning

	M	Tu	W	Th	F	Sa
Week #1 A.M.	1		3		2	
Week #1 P.M.		🌙		🌙		🌙
Week #2 A.M.	3		5		6	
Week #2 P.M.		🌙		1		🌙
Week #3 A.M.	7		1		8	6
Week #3 P.M.		9		🌙		
Week #4 A.M.	9		4		5	2
Week #4 P.M.		🌙		3		

Beginning Aquatic Programs

Aerobic endurance is your primary focus as you begin developing a new fitness program. Be sure to plan one full day of recovery after each workout, building up gradually until you are comfortable working at least four times a week in the Green and Blue zones. Workouts twice a day are especially beneficial if you are concentrating on reducing body fat. The more times you are active during the day, the higher your metabolism.

Moderate

	M	Tu	W	Th	F	Sa
Week #1 A.M.	2		7		1	10
Week #1 P.M.		2				
Week #2 A.M.	3		8		6	1
Week #2 P.M.				3		
Week #3 A.M.	4		5		4	
Week #3 P.M.		10		1		8
Week #4 A.M.	9		6		3	
Week #4 P.M.		5		2		3

Moderate Aquatic Programs

These schedules are geared toward those looking for muscle definition and major changes in their physical well-being. Having tried a few Green and Blue zone workouts, you've had the opportunity to learn how to work the water to your advantage. Whether it's streamlined strokes for laps or maximized resistance for vertical movements, this schedule should challenge you. Growth will come with one weekly workout that's one zone ahead of where you are currently working, in addition to your three basic workouts from the Purple and Yellow zones. Assign a high priority to maintaining your routine of regular workouts and you are on your way to minimizing the effects of aging and improving fitness.

Intense

	M	Tu	W	Th	F	Sa
Week #1 A.M.	9		5		4	
Week #1 P.M.		⟳		⟳	1	⟳
Week #2 A.M.	3	1	8		10	7
Week #2 P.M.				⟳		1
Week #3 A.M.	3	7		5	1	2
Week #3 P.M.			⟳			
Week #4 A.M.	10	5	8	5	2	4
Week #4 P.M.						

Intense Aquatic Programs

Strong muscles don't tire as quickly, so little recovery time is needed between laps or sets of exercises. You will use high-intensity, long-duration workouts back-to-back, but they will focus on different muscle groups each time. The variety of workouts in the Orange and Red zones will form the nucleus of your training schedule, using the first four zones for recovery days. This is a great time to try something new! Water puts everything in slow motion, making it easy to analyze techniques and acquire new skills without risk of injury. Every workout should be enjoyable and exhilarating. Find the combination of activities that best helps you maintain this fitness level.

Sequencing

After you have become familiar with the routines provided here, you may choose to supplement them with other favorite exercises. Try the human "cheat-sheet" to ensure that no body parts are left out. Visualize the human body and start at the top or bottom. Work each muscle group as you progress through the picture. Begin with the major muscle groups—smaller muscles fatigue quickly and won't be able to provide support for the larger moves if they are used first. Try to avoid doing many exercises that work the same muscle group back-to-back. Group enough large muscle moves together that you can receive cardiovascular conditioning for the minimum of 20 minutes. The shorter the rest between exercises, the greater the fitness benefits. While swimming laps, rest intervals of no more than 60 seconds are suggested.

14

Cross-Training

Enjoyed by high-level athletes because it reduces the chance of injury, cross-training employs more muscles, in a variety of ways. Cross-training simply means offering your body an occasional alternative form of exercise. We all become stale and risk injury with too much of a good thing. Choose alternating fitness activities that rate high in opposite areas. Refer to table 14.1 for ideas on activities that complement each other. Vertical aquatic fitness is a balanced and well-rounded activity, so any cross-training you choose will be a good complement. Swimming horizontally is 75 percent upper-body work, so cross-training in an activity focusing on the lower body complements the swimming. Fitness aquatics gives the body little or no impact, making high-impact activities like running or aerobic dance a nice match.

When you try a variety of activities, your body modifies its use of the nerve pathways and lever system. Greater muscle symmetry is likely to develop. The human body enjoys a challenge and the chance to react differently to different stimuli. Repeating one form of exercise exclusively may stress the same body parts, leading to overuse and possible injury. If you spread these stresses around the body to different joints and muscles, you can tolerate a higher volume of training.

Table 14.1
Complementary Cross-Training Choices

Activity	Impact	Focus	Strength	Flexibility	Cardiovascular	$	Calorie/Min. F	Calorie/Min. M
Cycling (9 mph)	Low	LB	2	1	3	$	5.6	7.4
Step aerobics	Mod	TB	2	2	3	$$	5.8	8.0
Rowing	Low	TB	3	3	3	$	6.6	7.6
Swimming	Low	UB	2	2	2	$	5	5.8
Golf	Low	UB	1	2	1	$$$	4.7	6.2
Deep-water running	None	TB	3	3	3	$	14.8	18.5
Tennis	High	TB	2	2	2	$$	6.2	8.3
Shallow-water exercise	Low	TB	3	3	3	$	14.6	18.1
Roller-blading	Low	LB	2	1	3	$	9.5	12.2
Yoga	Low	TB	2	3	1	$$		
Stair machine	Low	LB	2	1	3	$	8.8	11.6
Walking (3.5 mph)	Mod	LB	1	1	2	None	4.5	6.25
Dance aerobics	High	TB	2	3	3	$$	5.8	7.1
Weight training	Mod	TB	3	1	1	$	6.6	8.3
Soccer	High	LB	2	2	2	$	7.6	9.9
Volleyball	High	TB	1	2	1	$	2.8	4
Horseback riding	Mod	LB	1	1	1	$$$	4.3	5.2
Running	High	LB	2	1	3	$	11 10mm	15 6mm
Racquetball	High	TB	2	2	2	$$	7.6	10
Water skiing	Mod	TB	2	1	2	$$	6.2	9

3 = Excellent 2 = Good 1 = Poor   TB = Total body   UB = Upper body   LB = Lower body

Mentally, cross-training serves as a breath of fresh air. New surroundings or alternating days with different pieces of equipment keeps your mind alert. Feeling your muscles contract in minutely different ways can make exercise more fun. Many people drop exercise programs because they become bored with the repetition. Cross-training offers variety.

If you know a friend is waiting for you at the pool, you are less likely to roll over in bed and go back to sleep. This social factor is also a safety factor. When talking about bodies of water, remember to never enter alone! The most fit swimmers are just as susceptible to accidents and drowning as nonswimmers. Even if you think you'll just walk a few laps in the shallow end, at least have someone sit near the water and watch.

How Much is Enough?

It is common for many of my average clients to deep-water run for an hour and then water-box for a second hour. The focus of each class is very different. Just balance the workload over different muscles and cover a wide variety of activities. Working out three or four days a week usually works well for a person with an active lifestyle who aims to maintain a respectable level of fitness. If you have an inactive lifestyle, and no fitness plan, even one workout a week is an improvement.

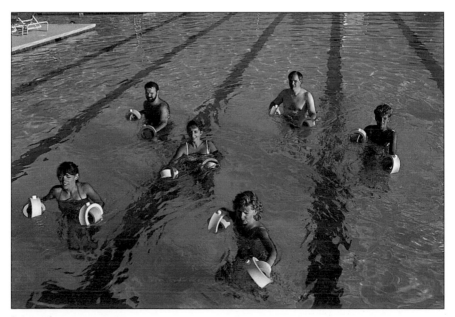

Join a class or a group.

Incorporate physical activities to add to your daily routine. Listen to your body. Feeling sleepy or running out of energy is often a plea for more oxygen or body heat, the kind derived through exercise, not a nap! Slowly add workouts to your weekly routine or increase their intensity. Always include an active rest day, or Green zone workout, to give the body time to rebuild and recover.

Table 14.2 Symptoms of Overtraining
Excessive fatigue
Stress fractures
Chronic pain
Anemia
Amenorrhea
Bursitis
Tendinitis
Elevated resting heart rate

Fitness cannot be stored. Overdoing it one week does not store up fitness points so you can take off the next week. Physical well-being disappears slowly with each week of disuse. It seems, however, that muscles have memories. Fitness returns faster for a person who was once fit than for a person who has never been fit.

Secrets to Successful Cross-Training

It takes a little extra effort to break from the security of an old routine, but the benefits are well worth it. Add one new activity at a time, waiting until you reach a respectable skill level before you add a new interest. Look for balance when you plan for cross-training week. Try to have alternative plans in case the pool shuts down or your bike has a flat. Once you call yourself a cross-trainer, there are no excuses for missing your workout!

Here are some suggestions for starting up:

- Devise a plan balancing all the components of fitness.
- Invest in appropriate gear and know how it is used.
- Approach new activities with respect.
- Have fun!

Re-Creating

Looking for a way to spice up even your favorite water workout? Try some tunes, explore a different pool, or teach someone what you've learned about water fitness. Try bright colors, a different center of buoyancy, a new technique to master. Review the equipment list in chapter 2 and treat yourself to a new toy. Create your own exercises. Travel through the water, change the timing, mix up arm and leg combinations to your heart's content.

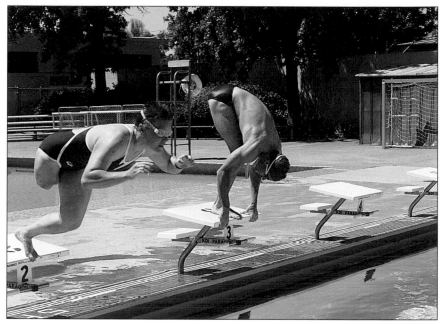

Aquatics is a great source of exercise for people with disabilities.

Monkey Around

Try performing a complete shallow-water workout in the shallow end without touching the bottom. Suspended! It will usually make an exercise more intense. Your arms will work harder and the hands will do a lot of sculling to keep you suspended. Chapter 4 also describes rebounding. If you have no medical reason to avoid impact, try an entire shallow-water workout getting your waist or hip bones out of the water each exercise. Land with your knee soft, ready for the next explosive move.

Music

Bring along your favorite cassette or CD with a snappy moderate beat. Use battery power, not electric power, near the water. Start the music and keep moving until it stops. Sing along if you know the words—you can develop your diaphragm at the same time. Select upbeat songs that make you want to move. All generations seem to be motivated by the John Phillip Sousa marches, and no toe can keep still with music from Herb Alpert and the Tijuana Brass.

Interval Training

Interval training combines high-intensity segments with moderate-to low-intensity segments. By using sets of varied intensity rather than prolonged repetitions, you can stay longer within your target heart rate or training zone and get an excellent cardiovascular workout. Intervals can be used at all levels of fitness. You can turn a workout from any of the zones into an interval workout, by adding a second set of each exercise. Alternate hard work and recovery work. Do the first set with all your might, then perform the second set in a relaxed fashion. Or try the first set small and tight and the second set slow and full-range. Many people use the 3:1 ratio. Start with three minutes at 60 percent to 75 percent MHR and give yourself one minute at 85 percent MHR. If that is easy, try a 2/2 split. As you get stronger, shorten the recovery time. Very advanced intervals will give you three minutes at high intensity and only a one-minute or 30-second recovery.

15

Charting Your Progress

Remember, the number-one reason people do not achieve success in their fitness goal is that they quit after just one or two workouts. If you have demonstrated your commitment by reading this book, buying water shoes, or investing in another piece of equipment, your chance of changing your level of fitness has improved from 60 percent to 80 percent. Evaluate your fitness level, choose the appropriate workout zones, and record your efforts in the progress chart in this chapter—now you have a 95 percent chance of improving your health.

Evaluating Performance Results

Making improvements in your fitness level is challenging and very rewarding. You will see results on the first day, when you prove to yourself how hard you can work and enjoy it. There will be no soreness the next day, but don't be fooled into thinking your workout was not productive. The water heals micro tears and increases circulation to carry away any toxins, so there is no soreness after exercise. Be consistent.

Exercising three days a week, you will notice physical changes in the small muscles within a few weeks. Changes in the larger muscles will soon follow. You sleep more soundly on the days you participate in water fitness. Your posture will improve and your energy level will rise.

If it's numbers that motivate you, keep your eye on your resting heart rate (RHR). As the heart muscle strengthens from regular conditioning it pumps fewer times to move the same volume of blood. RHR will decline over the months. Small increases in RHR day-to-day indicate you may be getting ill or you've been working too hard. Record your findings accurately and look at the big picture. The purpose of these numbers is to educate and motivate.

Goal Setting

The first step in setting goals was to test yourself. We will continually use those base numbers for comparison. Remember, though, you only compete with yourself. Your main goal is to maintain a consistent program. Many are thrilled to hold on to the status quo.

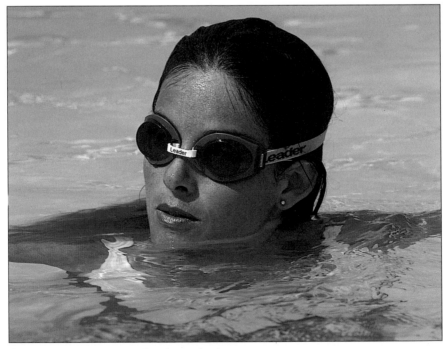

Once you've met your goals relax and enjoy.

© F-Stock/ David Stocklein

Be specific. Determine what it is you expect from a safe, effective exercise plan or what change needs to be made in your health. Break this idea down into specific tasks; for example, "I will plan for aerobic exercise three times a week" will keep you on track much better than "I'm going to start exercising this year." Better still, name a specific time and place, allowing yourself occasional flexibility.

Be realistic. You want your goals to be challenging but attainable. Increase any one F.I.T. principle by no more than 10 percent at a time, as suggested in chapter 1. Of course you will reset your goals often, but enjoy the sweet taste of success each time you complete an extra workout or try one in a more difficult zone.

Use short-term plans. Many people are overwhelmed with big projects and abandon them rather than actually fail. A goal like "I will lose 40 pounds this year" can seem overwhelming and restrictive at times. More success is found with goals like "I will keep my daily fat intake below 30 grams," or "I will eat to lose two pounds each week."

Lastly, take a few minutes to put your goals on paper. Put them in a place where you will see them often. Remind yourself of the original reason you chose that goal.

Sample Form

Month of: _____

Sunday	Monday	Tuesday	Wednesday	Thursday	Friday	Saturday	Weekly totals

Monthly total _____

Appendix

Suggested Aquatic Videos

Terrell Dougan
The Water Instructor's Home Companion
($25.00 + $5.00 S&H)
The Splash Co.
P.O. Box 58881
Salt Lake City, UT 84158-0881

Lynda Huey
Water Power Workout Video
($24.95 + $3.00 S&H)
Huey's Athletic Network
3014 Arizona Ave.
Santa Monica, CA 90404

Juliana Larson
Bounce Back Ability
($24.95 + $3.00 S&H)
Aquatic Networks
907 River Road, Ste. 202
Eugene, OR 97404

Equipment Distributors and Manufacturers

A.F.A. Aquatic Foam Accessories
P.O. Box 5752
Greenville, SC 29606
803 877-8428

Inventors of the Gyrojogger multi-use foot or hand flotation, Wet Wrap flotation belts, and Aqua blocks and bars with the built-in progress system.

AquaJogger Water Workout Gear
P.O. Box 5612
Eugene, OR 97405
800-922-9544

Heart rate monitors, belts, and a great tether that attaches to any flotation belt.

Art Di Rico Associates
4109 E. Parkway
Gatlinburg, TN 37738
615-436-5427

Suppliers of the Aqua Step and
the original Water Woggle.

Bioenergetics
2790 Montgomery Hwy.
Pelham, AL 35124
800-433-2627 or 214-350-1333

Makers of the Wet Vest I and II.
Designed for maximum comfort,
lift, and adjustability. Gloves,
belts, boots, and pillows are also
available.

D.K. Douglas Co., Inc.
299 Bliss Rd.
Longmeadow, MA 01106
800-334-9070

Thermal swimwear.

Gulbenkian Swimwear, Inc.
70 Memorial Plaza
Pleasantville, NY 10570
800-431-2586 Fax: 914-747-3243

Quality swimwear, specializing in
team and customized orders.

H₂O Works
c/o ERO Industries Inc.
585 Slawin Ct.
Mount Prospect, IL 60056-2183
800-323-5999

Products designed by an ortho-
pedic surgeon. H₂O Works provides swim mitts, tethers, flotation shorts, and a workout board
with flow-through design.

H₂Owear
1 Riverview Mill
P.O. Box 687
Wilton, NH 03086-0687

Aquatic fitnesswear for men and
women of all ages and abilities.
No suit lasts longer or feels more
comfortable.

**Hydro-Tone Fitness
Systems, Inc.**
16691 Gothard St., Ste. M
Huntington Beach, CA 92647
800-622-8663 Fax: 714-848-9035

Manufacturers of hand bells,
wave webs, flotation belts,
Hydro-Boots, and Hydro-Bells.

J&B Foam Fabricators
P.O. Box 144
Ludington, MI 49431
800-621-FOAM

J&B foam is easy to keep clean
and very long-lasting. Flotation
belts, water logs, and the greatest
kickboards ever made.

Land's End, Inc.
1 Land's End Lane
Dodgeville, WI 53595
800-356-4444 or 608-935-9341

Land's End has met the challenge
to provide water fitness
swimwear that stands up to chlo-
rine. Constructed of Lycra and
nylon to give all-way stretch,
these suits support, yet move
with every twist, stroke, and kick.

Index

About the Author

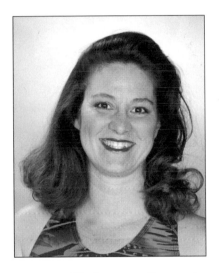

LeAnne Case, a master certified water fitness instructor, has taught individual and group exercise programs for people of all levels of fitness since 1980. As an aquatic fitness expert, she has certified hundreds of professional instructors.

Case has written numerous articles on aquatics training and travels around the world lecturing on the benefits of water fitness. The author is a member of Aquatic Alliance International (AAI), the Aquatic Exercise Association (AEA), and the United States Water Fitness Association (USWFA). She has served as National Technical Director for the USWFA, motivating and overseeing the work of nearly 50 instructors throughout the country.

Case received the North Carolina "Water Fitness Leader of the Year" award for 1993, 1994, and 1995. Through all her activities, she strives to expand knowledge of aquatic fitness techniques and effective methods of instruction.

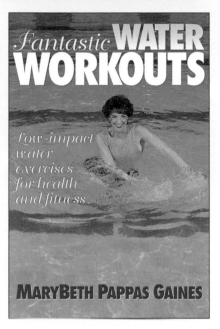
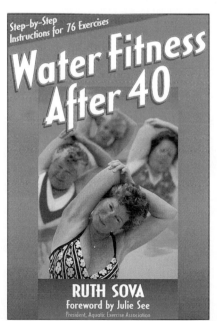